STAY **FIT** FOR LIFE

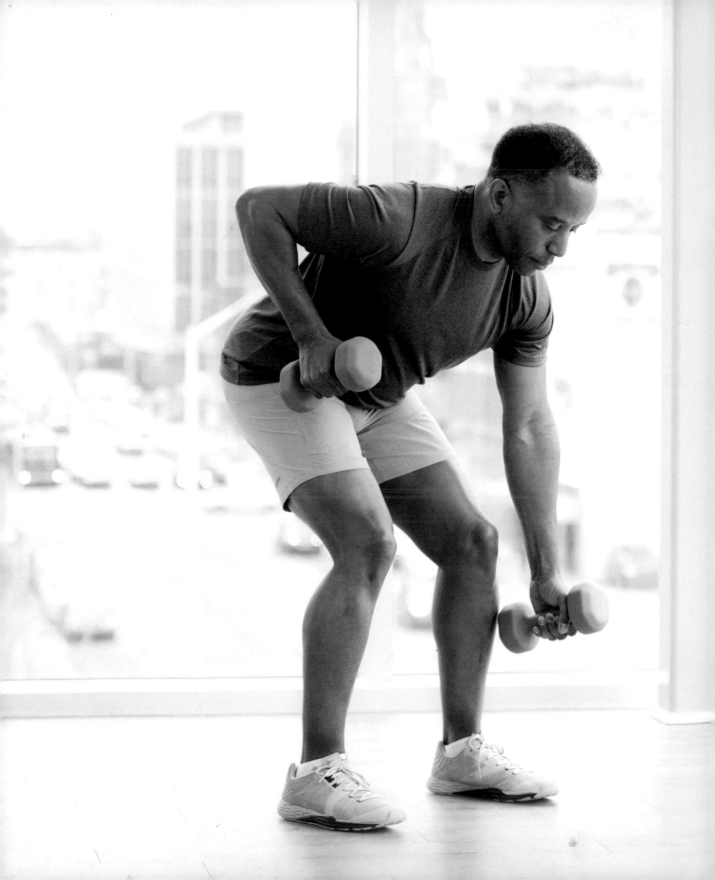

STAY
FIT
FOR
LIFE

JOSHUA KOZAK

Contents

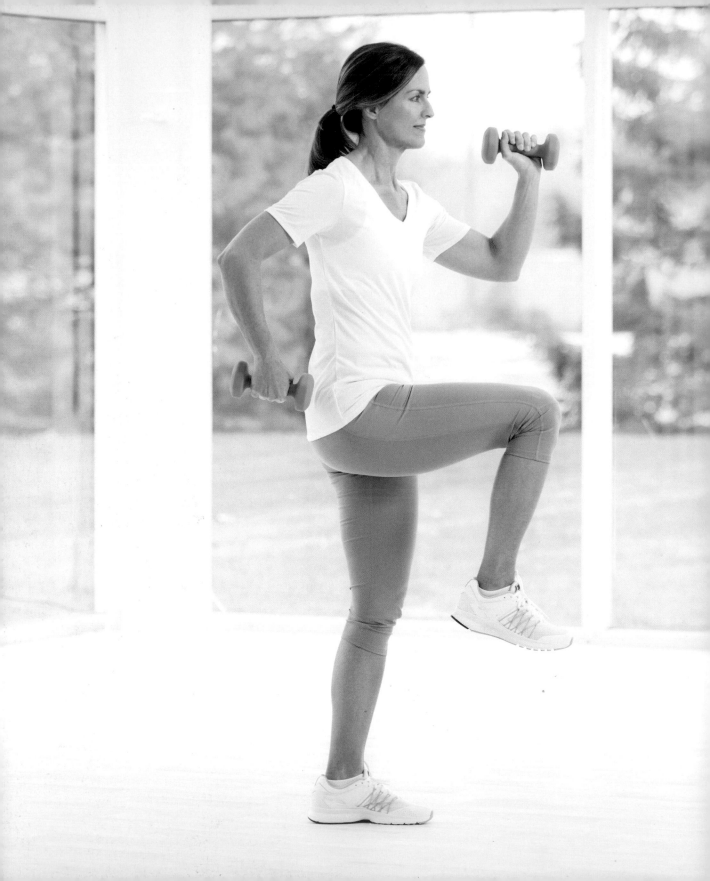

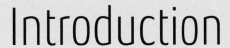

Introduction

We're all ageing, but not necessarily at the same rate. Have you ever wondered why one 70-year-old finds it difficult getting out of bed in the morning, while another is running half marathons? More often than not, it's because the marathon runner has kept all the parts of his or her body moving on a daily basis. That's what functional training is all about – engaging all parts of your body so you can still perform everyday activities with efficiency, no matter what your age.

So what is your goal? Maybe you want to be able to pick up your grandchildren with ease, start swimming again, or take those long walks you used to enjoy. Whatever it is, the moment you realize the direct correlation between improving your fitness and improving your life is the moment you will find all the motivation you need to stick to a fitness programme. The functional training method is the key to staying fit and active for life.

Use this book to future-proof your body with 62 step-by-step exercises (each with modifications to meet your ability level), 20 unique workout routines, and 3 easy-to-implement, one-month fitness programmes. *Stay Fit for Life* will empower you to do more of the things you love with confidence and ease for years to come.

FUNCTIONAL FITNESS BASICS

Functional training is a full-body approach to fitness that mimics your daily activities and enables you to live a healthier, more dynamic lifestyle. Life is unpredictable and unstable, so why should your training be full of predictable and stable movements?

Why train functionally?

By mimicking the way your body naturally moves, functional exercise strengthens your body's connections so you can move with ease and confidence, and continue to do the things you love as you age.

Prepare for daily life

Improving your body's efficiency through functional exercise lets you perform your daily activities more safely and substantially reduces your risk of injury as you age.

Improved posture

Functional training restores your body to its natural, upright state by improving flexibility in the spine, chest, and hips, while strengthening the back and glutes.

Greater strength

Strengthening your muscle groups makes it easier to perform daily tasks with more confidence and less pain. For example, functional training teaches your muscles to safely and effectively lift a heavy box.

Increased stability

Training your core with full-body movements improves balance and reduces the risk of falling. Strengthening the abdomen and back stabilizes your torso and gives you better control of your arms and legs.

Better mobility

Functional exercises enable you to move more freely and smoothly by increasing the range of motion of joints, improving flexibility, and helping you perform actions such as reaching and bending.

More endurance

Dynamic movements improve both cardiovascular and muscular endurance, which reduces your risk of developing chronic diseases, helps you control your weight, and preserves heart and lung health.

The benefits

Each exercise in this book tags the functional areas that it benefits in the Improves box. Follow a fitness programme to grow in all five areas.

IMPROVES

- Posture
- Strength
- Stability
- Mobility
- Endurance

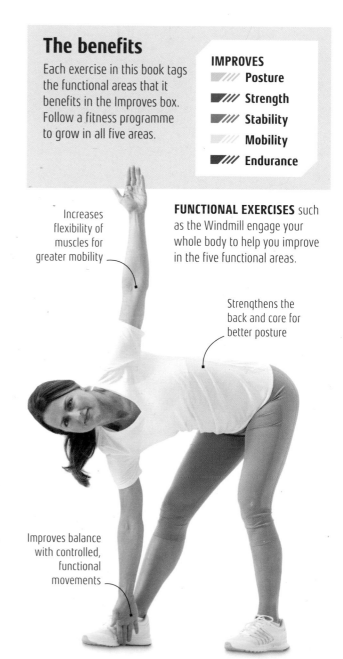

Increases flexibility of muscles for greater mobility

FUNCTIONAL EXERCISES such as the Windmill engage your whole body to help you improve in the five functional areas.

Strengthens the back and core for better posture

Improves balance with controlled, functional movements

The foundational movements

The human body can lift, flex, twist, and stretch in seemingly countless ways, but human movement can be distilled into five foundational types of movement: locomotion, pushing, pulling, rotation, and raising and lowering. Functional exercises require multiple joints and muscles to work together in the same way your everyday activities do, which improves your efficiency in these five movement patterns. A simple task such as picking up shopping bags involves your ankles, knees, hips, core, shoulders, and elbows; functional training mimics movements like this to help make everyday activities easier and safer to perform.

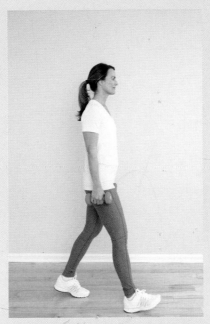

LOCOMOTION is the ability to move your body from one place to another. Activities such as walking, running, or climbing stairs all require locomotive skills.

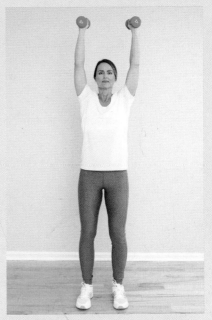

PUSHING involves activities that take your arms away from the body. Activities such as digging or moving a trolley full of shopping require efficient pushing.

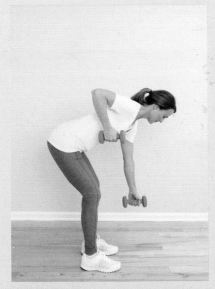

PULLING brings your arms towards your body or pulls your centre of mass towards an object. Examples include starting a lawn mower or pulling your chair up to a desk.

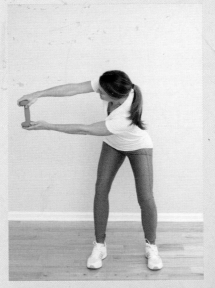

ROTATION requires the upper body to move in opposition to the lower body by twisting your hips and core. For example, swimming and throwing both use rotation.

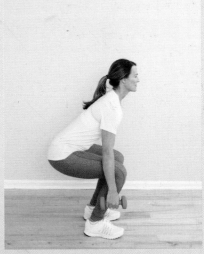

RAISING AND LOWERING the body's centre of mass involves bending, squatting, and lunging, and can be found in everyday tasks such as getting into a car.

How the body moves

Daily movement is dynamic, requiring a complex orchestration of your entire body in multiple directions and angles. Functional exercises use compound movements to train your body for that purpose. By understanding how your lower-body, core, and upper-body systems work together as one unit, you can move more efficiently and easily throughout your daily life.

Kinetic chain

Your individual muscles are useless without the kinetic chain – the body's system of joints, muscles, ligaments, and tendons that work together in a linear sequence to accomplish movement. For example, a throwing motion begins at your ankles and transfers force through the kinetic chain all the way to your wrists. Some links in the chain keep your joints stable, while others enable mobility; but if one link is not working properly, it will affect surrounding links, and ultimately the movement.

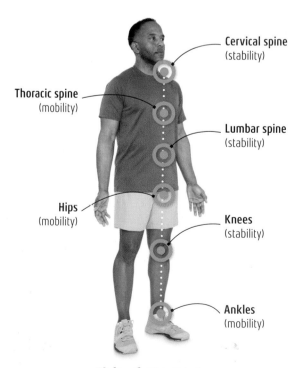

Cervical spine
(stability)

Thoracic spine
(mobility)

Lumbar spine
(stability)

Hips
(mobility)

Knees
(stability)

Ankles
(mobility)

Links of movement

Planes of movement

Your body moves within three dimensions, called planes. If you imagine all the different movements your body can make, every one of them occupies at least one plane of movement. However, most actions are not performed precisely in one plane, but rather they use multiple planes at once – we move up and down and side to side in fluid motions. Functional training works your body in all 3 planes of movement to improve overall coordination and stability.

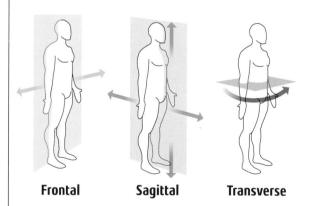

Frontal   **Sagittal**   **Transverse**

FRONTAL PLANE divides the front and back halves of the body. We move from side to side in this plane.

SAGITTAL PLANE splits the left and right sides of the body. We move up and down or forwards and backwards in this plane.

TRANSVERSE PLANE separates the top and bottom of the body at the hips. We rotate in this plane.

Compound exercise

Functional exercises are usually compound, meaning they use several muscle groups at once. By performing exercises that recruit your whole kinetic chain within multiple planes of movement, you effectively prepare your body for any movement challenge that an active life may throw your way.

A COMPOUND MOVEMENT, such as the Reverse lunge with twist, can use multiple planes of movement (the transverse and saggital planes, in this instance), while engaging the total kinetic chain.

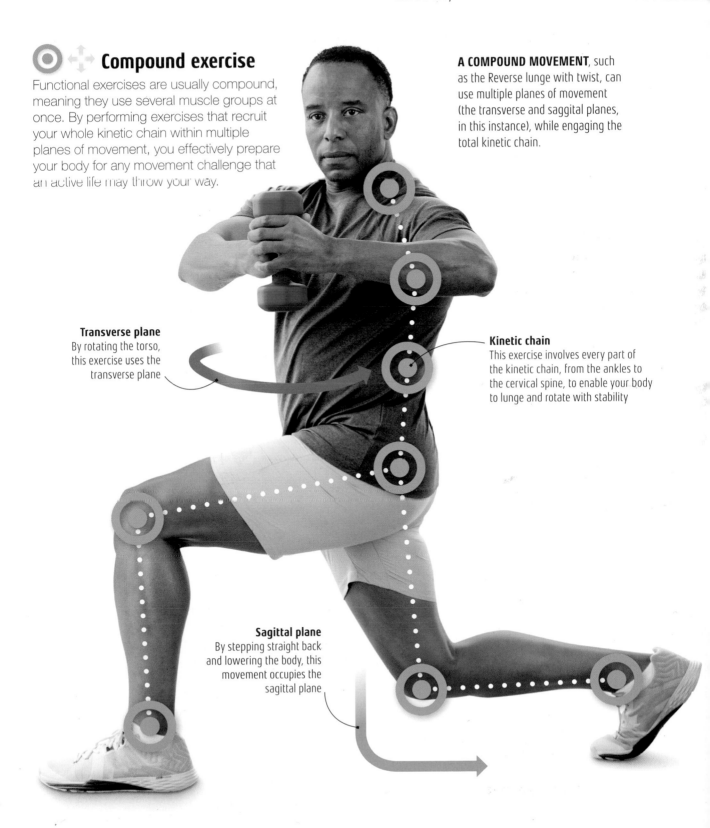

Transverse plane
By rotating the torso, this exercise uses the transverse plane

Kinetic chain
This exercise involves every part of the kinetic chain, from the ankles to the cervical spine, to enable your body to lunge and rotate with stability

Sagittal plane
By stepping straight back and lowering the body, this movement occupies the sagittal plane

How exercise helps the body

You've probably heard the axiom "move it or lose it", and it's true. Nothing will speed up the ageing process quite like disuse and inactivity of the body, but performing functional exercise on a regular basis will improve your health and quality of life, and keep your body looking and feeling youthful.

STRENGTHENS BONES

1% Amount of bone density the average person loses each year after age **35**

Bones tend to weaken with age, but functional training uses weight-bearing exercises to slow down bone-density loss. By loading your bones with weight, you increase muscle mass, which is proven to directly increase bone cell growth and help prevent osteoporosis and fractures.

BUILDS LEAN MUSCLE

4% Amount of muscle mass the average person loses each decade after age **30**

With age and inactivity, the body can experience a significant loss of muscle mass, a condition called *muscle atrophy*. However, when you perform weight-bearing exercises, your body replaces damaged muscle fibres with new fibres that strengthen and build lean muscle tissue. Stronger muscles enable you to live a more confident and active lifestyle.

PRESERVES VITAL JOINT TISSUES

350 million

Estimated number of people worldwide who have arthritis

The breakdown of joint tissue over time can lead to pain, inflammation, stiffness, and often arthritis. Functional exercise stimulates blood flow to joint tissues so that the increased supply of oxygen and nutrients can lubricate your joints. This results in healthier, pain-free movement.

SHARPENS NERVOUS SYSTEM

3.4 million

Number of people over **65** who suffer from a fall in the UK each year

Your nervous system and brain function inevitably decline with age, which impairs your ability to sense your body's movement and position in space – known as *proprioception*. Functional training focuses on movements that build a strong connection between your brain and body to improve your proprioception, and increase your reaction time, for safer and more agile movement.

IMPROVES HEART HEALTH AND BLOOD FLOW

31 % Percentage of total deaths worldwide in **2015** due to heart disease

An ageing heart can't pump out as much blood as a younger heart, but functional fitness boosts your heart's endurance, lowers your resting heart rate, and causes blood vessels to dilate, which means more oxygen reaches your organs and muscles. Increased flow of oxygen gives you the energy to move with more vitality.

IMPROVES MOOD AND CONFIDENCE

350 million

Number of people worldwide who suffer from depression

When you're stressed, your body releases stress hormones, such as cortisol and adrenaline, that can produce inflammation in your body and lead to anxiety and depression. Functional training combats this by engaging your body to release feel-good hormones, or *endorphins*, that counter the negative effects of stress and anxiety to lift your mood and increase your confidence.

EXTENDS LIFE SPAN

7 minutes

Length of time your life is extended by every minute of exercise after age **39**

Study after study has shown that a sedentary lifestyle can have devastating effects on individual health, including a shortened life span. Functional training helps rebuild and re-energize weakened muscles and joints, strengthens the heart and lungs, and improves and extends your life. The benefit may level off as you age, but when you give a little, you always gain a little. It's never too late to start, so get moving!

INCREASES LUNG FUNCTION

1/3 Amount a person's lung capacity reduces from age **30** to **60**

The effects of ageing on the respiratory system include weakened lungs and respiratory muscles, making you feel short of breath when you exercise. But increased fitness levels make your movement and heart more efficient, thus making it easier for your lungs to supply your body with oxygen. You'll notice increased stamina the more you work out.

BOOSTS METABOLISM

2% Amount a person's metabolism slows with each decade of life

Your basal metabolic rate (BMR) is the number of calories your body burns at rest. Functional training increases your BMR by increasing your lean muscle mass. Because muscle cells require energy in the form of calories, even when you're not exercising, increasing your muscle mass makes your body more efficient at burning calories to keep you leaner.

How to train effectively

Getting fit doesn't require spending long hours at the gym, but it does require taking good care of your body and observing some essential rules for effective training and living. To get the most out of your training, begin building healthy habits and follow this exercise and lifestyle guidance.

Q HOW MUCH WATER SHOULD I DRINK EVERY DAY?

A You should drink 2 litres of water, or about eight glasses, every day. Staying hydrated helps your heart and muscles work more efficiently. Drink water before the thirst sensation even arises – if you're already thirsty, then you're already dehydrated. It helps to carry a water bottle with you everywhere you go so you can drink throughout the day.

Q HOW DO I KNOW IF I'M DEHYDRATED?

A Listen to your body. Thirst, headaches, dizziness, and fatigue are all potential signs of dehydration. If you feel any of these symptoms, then it's possible you need more water. Urine colour is also a good indicator. Ideally it's a pale straw colour, but if it is dark yellow, then you're likely to be dehydrated. On the other hand, colourless urine might mean you're over-hydrated or drinking too quickly.

Q SHOULD I EAT BEFORE WORKING OUT?

A Yes! Eat a nutrient-rich meal between 1 and 3 hours before training. Eating before a workout provides essential nutrients to increase the effectiveness of your hard work. Whole foods are best – primarily low-fat proteins and low-glycemic carbohydrates such as eggs, oats, chicken, and vegetables.

Q WHEN SHOULD I EAT AFTER WORKING OUT?

A Eat a post-workout meal within 15 to 20 minutes after working out. This meal should consist of a 3:1 ratio of carbohydrates to proteins to give your muscles the fuel to replenish glycogen, a substance that rebuilds and repairs muscle tissues. Good meal options include fish and brown rice, or turkey and sweet potatoes.

Q HOW CAN I SHOP SMARTER?

A Shop the perimeter of the supermarket and avoid centre aisles. The perimeter of most shops is where you'll find whole foods, fruits and vegetables, dairy, and lean meats. By comparison, the centre aisles tend to be where high-sugar and highly-processed foods are shelved. By avoiding centre aisles, it is easier to fill your trolley with healthy fuel options.

Q HOW SHOULD I BREATHE WHILE I'M EXERCISING?

A You should exhale through your mouth during the hardest part of a movement and inhale through your nose during the easier part, keeping a steady, mindful rhythm. Using a squat as an example, inhale on the way down and then exhale as you stand up. However, don't worry too much about exactly when to breathe – the most important thing is to remember not to hold your breath.

Q DO I REALLY NEED TO COOL DOWN AFTER A WORKOUT?

A Absolutely. It's essential to cool down at a controlled pace after every workout. After training, your heart rate is high, your blood vessels are dilated, and your body temperature is elevated. Stopping too fast can lead to passing out or feeling sick. Steadily slowing down lets your body comfortably transition back to a state of rest.

Q HOW CAN I LIMIT SORENESS AFTER TRAINING?

A Integrate foam rolling into your post-workout regime. The sustained pressure to your muscle tissues deeply lengthens them, ensures they don't tighten up too quickly after exercise, and increases the range of motion of your joints. Use this method to release any of your soft tissues – including your glutes, thighs, calves, chest, or upper back – but never roll over bones or organs.

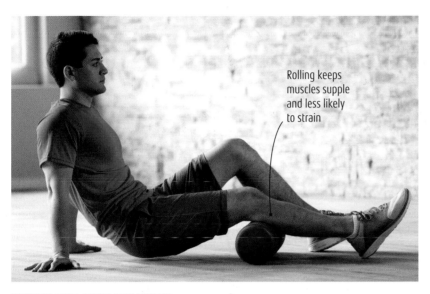

Rolling keeps muscles supple and less likely to strain

SLOWLY ROLL BACK AND FORTH over your soft tissues, applying pressure with body weight, for about 30 seconds.

Q DO I HAVE TO WORK OUT EVERY DAY?

A No. Your mind and body need time to recover, so always include two rest days during your exercise week. When you don't take your rest days, it can lead to mental burnout and an inability to sustain your fitness progress and achieve your goals. Time off also allows your muscles to relax and rebuild, which will make you stronger and less prone to injury. If you're feeling overly tired, or if your muscles and joints feel excessively stiff, it's a good time to take a rest day.

What does it take to stay fit for life?

Breathe consciously, even at rest

Breathing is so involuntary that some people are never really conscious of it until their bodies are starved of oxygen, such as during exercise. However, breathing deeply and deliberately – even while you're at rest – can improve your brain function, relax your body, and reduce stress.

Get quality sleep every night

Sleep is when your mind and body heal and recharge, so it is essential for a healthy lifestyle. Try to get 7 to 8 hours of quality sleep each night. For a more restful sleep, avoid drinking alcohol or large amounts of liquid at least two hours before bedtime, and try to go to bed at the same time each night.

Make time to exercise

It's easy to put off a workout, so always plan exactly when you'll do your workout routine, and try to make it consistent each day. A steady schedule helps you stay on track and ensures that you'll stick to your plan.

Be your own best coach

It's easy to stay motivated when you're in a groove, but it's normal to get off track sometimes. If you find yourself avoiding the gym or straying from a programme, stay positive, don't be too hard on yourself, and go back to where you left off. Usually just completing that next workout is enough to help you regain lost momentum.

How to use this book

Stay Fit for Life is comprised of a collection of individual exercises, daily workout routines, and functional training programmes that will help you get stronger and healthier. This simple method takes the guesswork out of your fitness regime. Start by performing the fitness assessment, and the rest will fall into place – all you need is the motivation to stick with it.

1 >> PERFORM THE ASSESSMENT TESTS

Perform each of the five assessment tests on the following pages and use your scores to calculate your fitness level: beginner, intermediate, or advanced. This tells you which exercise programme to follow to get started with your training.

Score yourself on a scale of 1–4 for each test

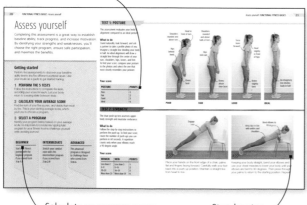

Calculate an average score that will tell you which of the 3 programmes to use

Step-by-step pictures show how to perform the tests

2 >> FIND YOUR FITNESS PROGRAMME

Identify your fitness programme based on your assessment results. Each 30-day programme progresses in difficulty throughout the course of four weeks. The simple calendar design shows you exactly what to do each day.

Workout days specify the prescribed routine for that day, as well as which level to follow

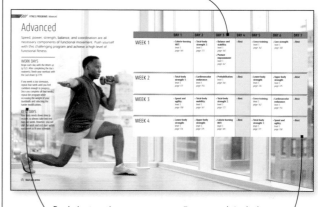

Basic instructions explain how to work through the programmes

Every week includes rest days, which are essential for rejuvenating your body

What you need

Only a few simple pieces of equipment are
needed to perform the exercises
in this book.

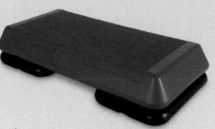

Dumbbells
These help you get the most out of your exercise. We
recommend having two pairs, one lighter and one heavier,
so you can adjust the weight for difficulty.

Step
An aerobic step
is used in some
cardio and strength
exercises. A stair or low
bench works well, too.

Mat
An exercise mat makes floor-based exercises more comfortable.

Chair
Use a sturdy, non-slip chair for some bodyweight exercises, for
support to help you balance, or to do a movement while seated.

3 >>> TURN TO THE DAILY WORKOUT ROUTINE

Find your assigned workout for the day, and identify
the level prescribed by your programme. Each
workout routine is composed of five to ten individual
exercises that work towards the routine's goal. Follow
the directions to complete your level of the workout.

Purposefully chosen
exercises work together
to help you achieve each
workout's goal

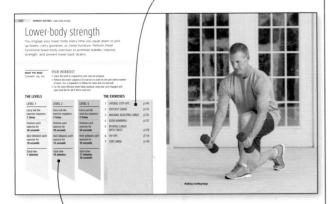

The level shows you how long
to perform each exercise, then
how long to rest between
each exercise

4 >>> COMPLETE THE REQUIRED EXERCISES

Refer to the step-by-step instruction pages to help
you execute the exercises in your workout. Each of
the 62 exercises found in the routines has its own
highly visual spread showing you how to perform
the exercise using proper technique.

Each spread identifies
which of the five
foundational movements
the exercise engages

Helpful annotations
provide tips for
performing the
exercise correctly

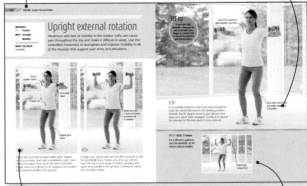

Detailed, step-by-step
instructions and colour photos
show you exactly how to
perform the exercise from
start to finish

Whenever you want to
make an exercise easier
or more challenging,
follow the directions for
the modifications

Assess yourself

Completing this assessment is a great way to establish baseline ability, track progress, and increase motivation. By identifying your strengths and weaknesses, you'll choose the right programme, ensure safe participation, and maximize the benefits.

Getting started

Perform the assessments to discover your baseline ability level in the five different functional areas. Use your results as a guide to get started training.

1 PERFORM THE 5 TESTS
Follow the instructions to complete the tests, recording your score for each. Let your body return to a resting state between tests.

2 CALCULATE YOUR AVERAGE SCORE
Find the sum of your five scores, and divide that result by five. This is your starting average score, which you'll use to choose a programme.

3 SELECT A PROGRAMME
Identify your programme below based on your average score. It's important to choose the appropriate programme for your fitness level to challenge yourself while avoiding burnout.

BEGINNER
Start your fitness journey with the beginner programme if you scored from **1 to 1.9**

INTERMEDIATE
Stretch your comfort zone with this programme if you scored from **2 to 2.9**

ADVANCED
The advanced programme is designed to challenge those who scored from **3 to 4**

TEST 1: POSTURE

This assessment evaluates your body's alignment compared to an ideal posture.

What to do
Stand naturally, look forward, and ask a partner to take a profile photo of you. Imagine a straight line dividing your body in half. An ideal alignment will draw a straight line through the centre of your ears, shoulders, hips, knees, and feet. To find your score, compare your posture to the photos and select the one that most closely resembles your posture.

Your score

POSTURE	POINTS
Poor	1
Fair	2
Good	3
Ideal	4

TEST 2: STRENGTH

The chair push-up test assesses upper-body strength and muscular endurance.

What to do
Follow the step-by-step instructions to perform the push-up. To find your score, count the number of push-ups you can perform in 60 seconds. A repetition counts only when your elbows reach a 90-degree angle.

Your score

WOMEN	MEN	POINTS
Less than 2	Less than 5	1
3–9	5–15	2
10–25	16–35	3
More than 25	More than 35	4

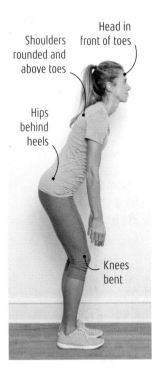

Shoulders rounded and above toes

Head in front of toes

Hips behind heels

Knees bent

POOR

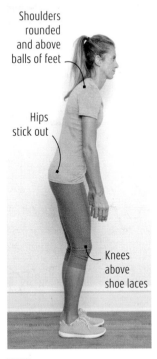

Shoulders rounded and above balls of feet

Hips stick out

Knees above shoe laces

FAIR

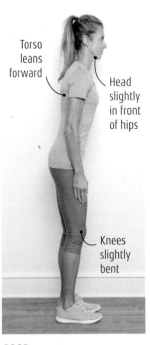

Torso leans forward

Head slightly in front of hips

Knees slightly bent

GOOD

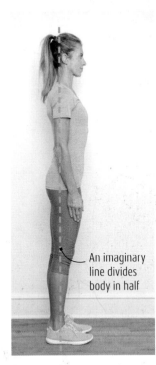

An imaginary line divides body in half

IDEAL

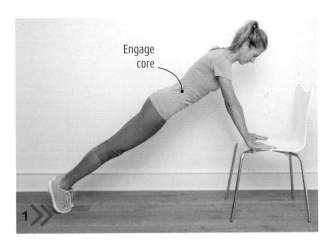

Engage core

Place your hands on the front edge of a chair, palms flat and fingers facing forward. Carefully walk your feet back into a push-up position. Maintain a straight line from head to toe.

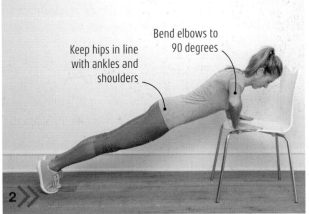

Keep hips in line with ankles and shoulders

Bend elbows to 90 degrees

Keeping your body straight, bend your elbows and use your chest muscles to lower your body until your elbows are bent to 90 degrees. Then press through your palms to return to the starting position. Repeat.

TEST 3: STABILITY

Use this test to evaluate your balance and stability while in a static position.

What to do
Follow the step-by-step instructions to get into position. Using a stopwatch, time how long you can balance on your left leg before your right foot touches the ground. Repeat on your right leg. To find your score, calculate the average of your two times.

Your score

ALL	POINTS
Less than 20 seconds	1
21–35 seconds	2
36–50 seconds	3
More than 50 seconds	4

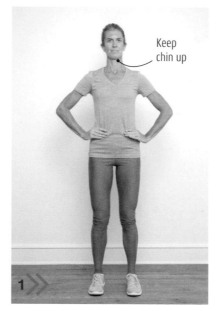

Keep chin up

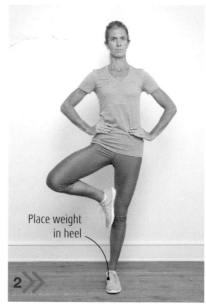

Place weight in heel

1 ≫ Stand with your feet shoulder-width apart and place your hands on your hips. Maintain an upright posture and engage your core. Retract your shoulder blades.

2 ≫ Lift your right leg and place the sole of the right foot against the side of your left knee. Time how long you can balance in this position. Repeat on your other leg.

TEST 5: MOBILITY

The overhead squat tests your flexibility and mobility on both sides of the body.

What to do
Stand with your feet shoulder-width apart and raise your arms straight overhead. Squat as deeply as you can, and ask a partner to take a profile photo of you. To find your score, select the photo that most closely resembles your position.

Your score

POSITION	POINTS
Poor	1
Fair	2
Good	3
Ideal	4

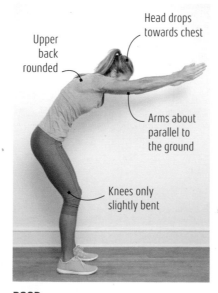

Upper back rounded

Head drops towards chest

Arms about parallel to the ground

Knees only slightly bent

POOR

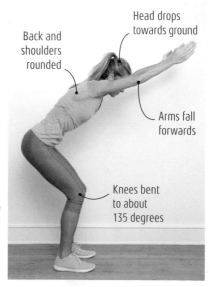

Back and shoulders rounded

Head drops towards ground

Arms fall forwards

Knees bent to about 135 degrees

FAIR

TEST 4: ENDURANCE

This step test assesses your cardiovascular endurance.

What to do

Follow the step-by-step instructions. To find your score, count the number of times your left knee reaches the mark in 2 minutes.

Your score

WOMEN	POINTS
Less than 80	1
81–100	2
101–120	3
More than 120	4

MEN	POINTS
Less than 90	1
91–110	2
111–130	3
More than 130	4

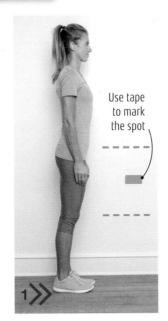

Use tape to mark the spot

1 » Stand next to a wall and mark the spot that is halfway between your hip bone and knee.

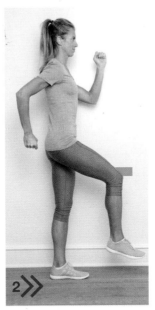

2 » Lift your right knee until it reaches the mark on the wall. Swing your arms to help balance.

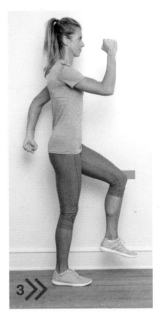

3 » Lower your right leg to the ground, then raise your left knee to the mark. Continue to march in place.

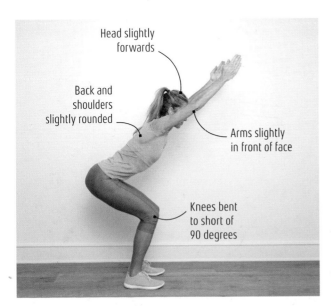

Head slightly forwards

Back and shoulders slightly rounded

Arms slightly in front of face

Knees bent to short of 90 degrees

GOOD

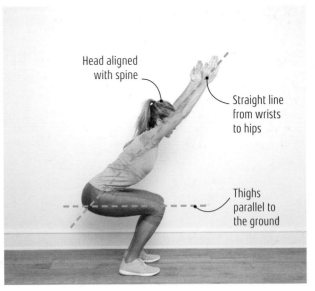

Head aligned with spine

Straight line from wrists to hips

Thighs parallel to the ground

IDEAL

EXERCISES

LOCOMOTION • PUSHING • PULLING • ROTATION • RAISING AND LOWERING

Living an active lifestyle requires a wide range of movements, so it is important to be prepared. By targeting your body's five foundational movements, this collection of functional exercises will make you stronger, more stable, and better equipped to tackle your everyday activities.

Fast feet

IMPROVES
/// **Endurance**

WHAT YOU NEED
No equipment needed

Strong communication between your brain and body is the key to moving quickly during walking activities. Run in place with this drill to improve your mind-body coordination and cardiovascular endurance.

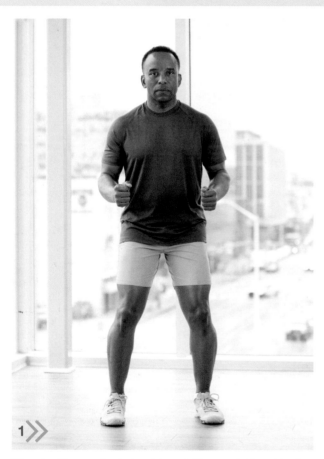

1 >>

Stand with your feet shoulder-width apart. Bend both elbows to 90 degrees, position your forearms in front of you, and hold your hands in loose fists. Engage your core and retract your shoulder blades.

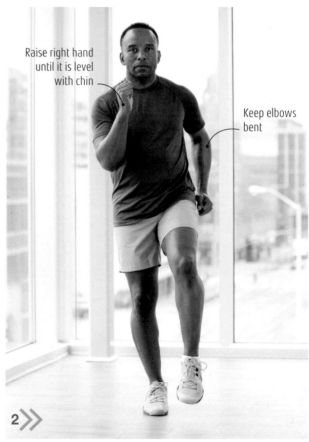

Raise right hand until it is level with chin

Keep elbows bent

2 >>

Raise your left knee until your foot is about 8cm (3in) off the ground, and shift your weight to your right foot. Simultaneously raise your right hand towards your chin and pull your left hand towards your hip.

3 »

In a continuous motion, return your left foot to the ground, first making contact with the ball of your foot, and immediately lift your right foot about 8cm (3in) off the ground while raising your left hand towards your chin and pulling your right hand towards your hip. Continue to run in place for the time given in your workout.

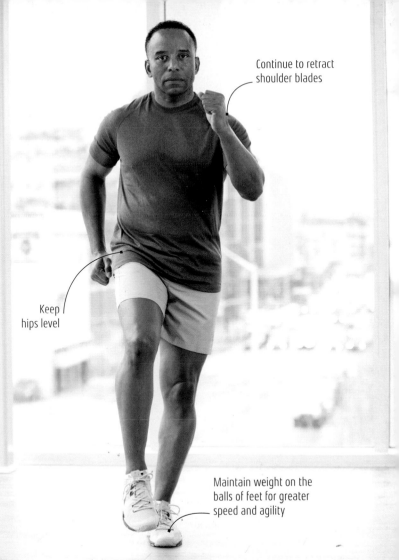

Continue to retract shoulder blades

Keep hips level

Maintain weight on the balls of feet for greater speed and agility

//// MAKE IT **easier**

If it is difficult to maintain balance, sit on the edge of a chair and run in place while seated.

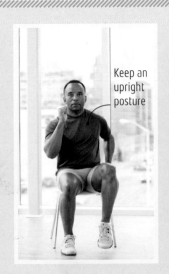

Keep an upright posture

//// MAKE IT **harder**

To increase intensity, raise your knee as high as you can with each step.

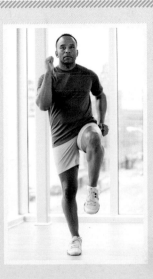

IMPROVES
▰/// **Stability**
▰/// **Endurance**

WHAT YOU NEED
No equipment needed

Side-to-side

Because life tasks often require you to move sideways, lateral exercises such as this one are essential to any fitness programme. This fast-paced drill enhances your stability and coordination so you can move left and right with confidence.

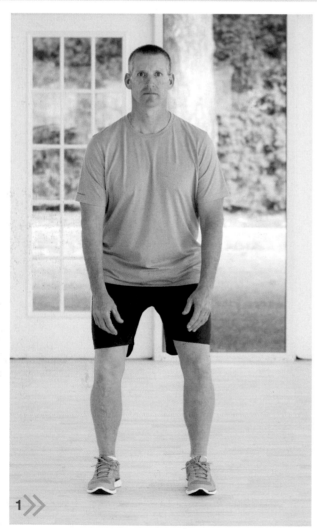

1 ⟫

Stand with your feet shoulder-width apart and relax your arms in front of you. Engage your core, slightly lean forwards, retract your shoulder blades, and raise your head. Slightly bend your knees and hips.

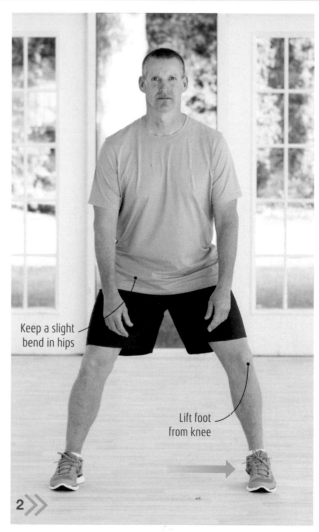

Keep a slight bend in hips

Lift foot from knee

2 ⟫

Raise your left foot off the ground and step to your left, first making contact with the ball of your foot, then with your heel. Step out slightly wider than shoulder-width apart.

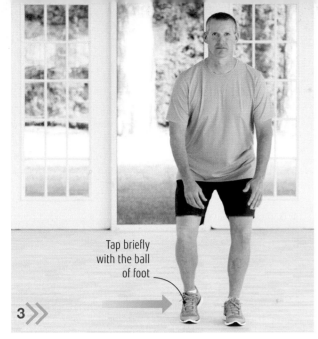

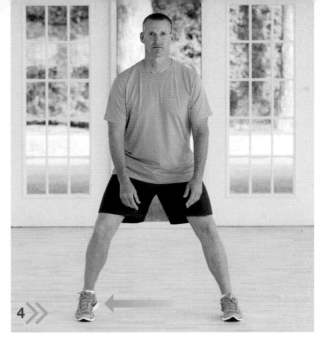

3 ›› Raise your right foot off the ground and tap it next to your left foot, transferring your weight to your left foot. Make light and brief contact with the ball of your right foot, and do not place your heel on the ground.

Tap briefly with the ball of foot

4 ›› Quickly step your right foot back to slightly wider than shoulder-width apart and shift your weight back to your right foot. Maintain a slight bend in your knees and hips for balance.

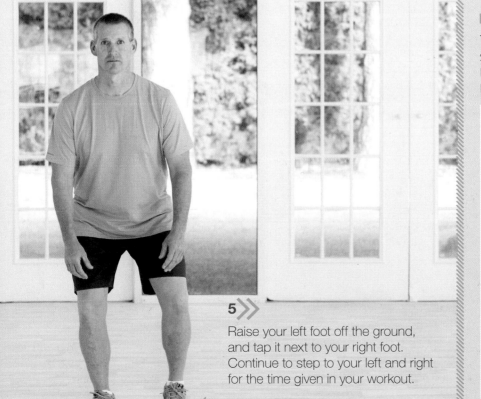

5 ›› Raise your left foot off the ground, and tap it next to your right foot. Continue to step to your left and right for the time given in your workout.

//// **MAKE IT harder**

To strengthen your legs, in step 1, squat until your thighs are parallel to the ground. Maintain the squat throughout the exercise.

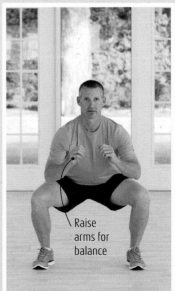

Raise arms for balance

Side shuffle

Lateral movements require agility, coordination, and stability. Shuffling quickly from side to side will improve your ability to perform these sideways motions while also strengthening your legs and glutes.

IMPROVES

■/// **Strength**

■/// **Stability**

■/// **Endurance**

WHAT YOU NEED

No equipment needed

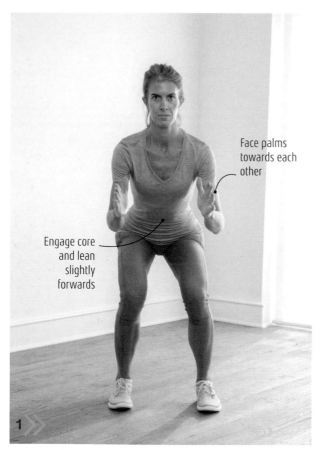

Face palms towards each other

Engage core and lean slightly forwards

1

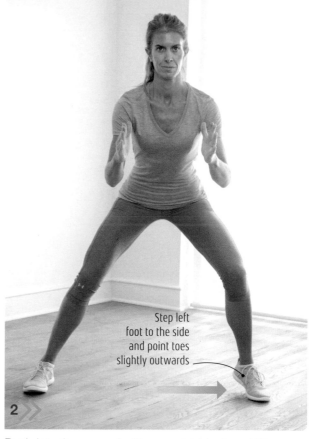

Step left foot to the side and point toes slightly outwards

2

Stand with your feet shoulder-width apart and bend your knees and hips. Place your weight in your hips and heels. Raise your head and retract your shoulder blades. Hold your arms firmly in front of you.

Push into the ground with your right foot and lift your left foot off the ground. Step to your left and place your left foot wider than shoulder-width apart. Transfer your weight to your left foot.

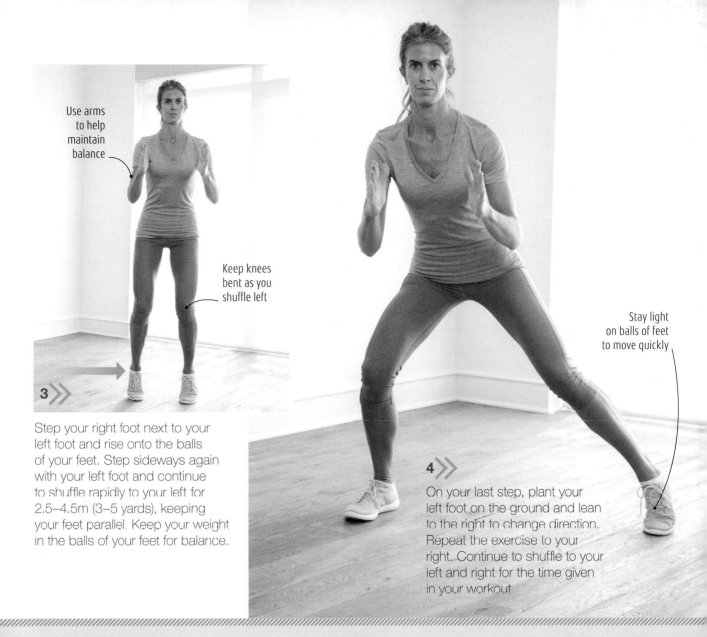

Use arms to help maintain balance

Keep knees bent as you shuffle left

Stay light on balls of feet to move quickly

3 »

Step your right foot next to your left foot and rise onto the balls of your feet. Step sideways again with your left foot and continue to shuffle rapidly to your left for 2.5–4.5m (3–5 yards), keeping your feet parallel. Keep your weight in the balls of your feet for balance.

4 »

On your last step, plant your left foot on the ground and lean to the right to change direction. Repeat the exercise to your right. Continue to shuffle to your left and right for the time given in your workout.

///// MAKE IT harder

To strengthen your legs, in step 1, squat deep until your thighs are parallel to the ground. Maintain the squat throughout the exercise.

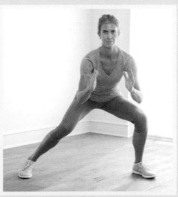

March in place

IMPROVES

/// **Stability**

/// **Mobility**

/// **Endurance**

WHAT YOU NEED
No equipment needed

Running, hiking, and climbing stairs all demand your hips be flexible and strong. Perform this drill energetically to improve your endurance and balance while stretching and strengthening your hips.

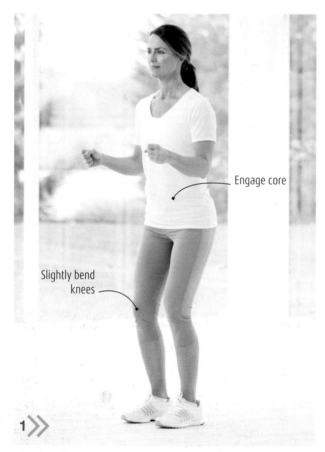

Engage core

Slightly bend knees

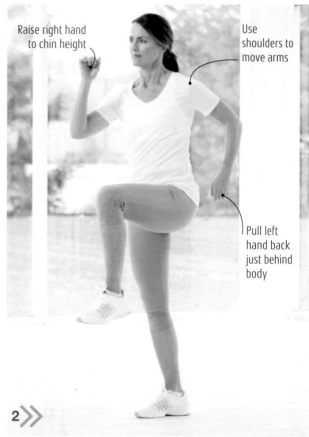

Raise right hand to chin height

Use shoulders to move arms

Pull left hand back just behind body

1 »
Stand with your feet shoulder-width apart. Bend both elbows to 90 degrees, position your forearms in front of you, and hold your hands in loose fists. Lengthen your spine and retract your shoulder blades.

2 »
Shift your weight to your right foot and raise your left knee until your thigh is parallel to the ground. Simultaneously swing your right arm up and your left arm back, maintaining the bend in your elbows.

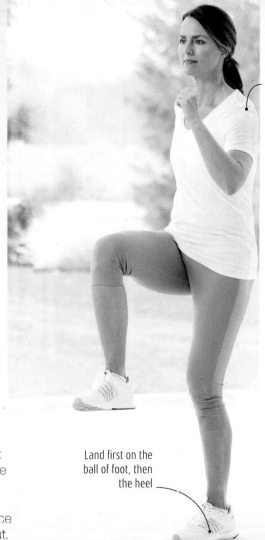

Maintain an upright posture

3 »

Quickly return your left foot to the ground and shift your weight to your left foot. Immediately raise your right knee and swing your arms in the opposite directions. Continue to march rapidly in place for the time given in your workout.

Land first on the ball of foot, then the heel

///// **MAKE IT** easier

If it is difficult to maintain balance, sit on the edge of a chair and do the exercise by raising your feet about 15cm (6in) from the ground.

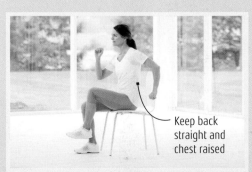

Keep back straight and chest raised

///// **MAKE IT** harder

To strengthen your shoulders, hold a dumbbell in each hand as you do the exercise.

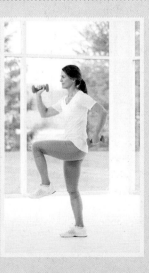

High knee and reach

Perform this energy-intensive, total-body reach quickly to improve your stamina and stability. By dynamically engaging multiple muscle groups, you increase your body's endurance for powerful movement.

IMPROVES

▰/// **Stability**

/// **Mobility**

▰/// **Endurance**

WHAT YOU NEED
No equipment needed

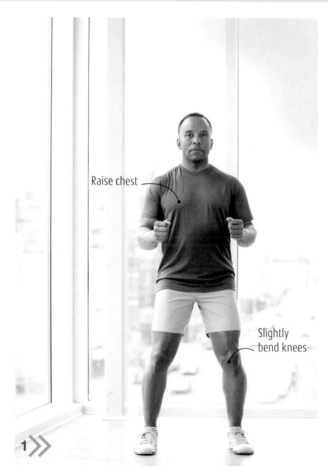

Raise chest

Slightly bend knees

1 ≫

Stand with your feet shoulder-width apart. Bend both elbows to 90 degrees, position your forearms in front of you, and hold your hands in loose fists. Engage your core and retract your shoulder blades.

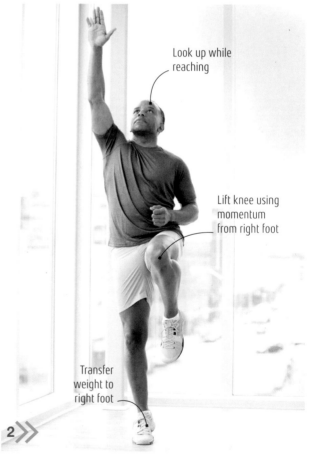

Look up while reaching

Lift knee using momentum from right foot

Transfer weight to right foot

2 ≫

Powerfully rise onto the ball of your right foot, letting your heel come off the ground, and raise your left knee until your thigh is parallel to the ground. Simultaneously reach overhead with your right hand as if you are grabbing something from a high shelf.

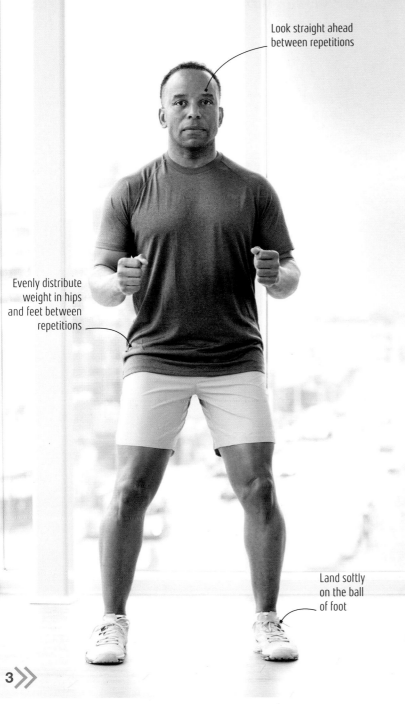

Look straight ahead
between repetitions

Evenly distribute
weight in hips
and feet between
repetitions

Land softly
on the ball
of foot

3 »

Lower both feet and your right arm to the starting position,
and slightly bend your knees to absorb your weight. Quickly
repeat the exercise by rising onto the ball of your left foot
and raising your right knee and left hand. Alternate rapidly
on each side for the time given in your workout.

MAKE IT **easier**

If it is difficult to maintain
balance, sit on the edge of a chair
and do the exercise by raising
your feet about 7cm (3in) from
the ground.

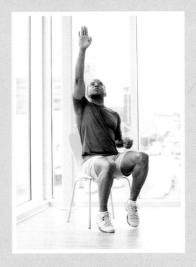

MAKE IT **harder**

To increase intensity, in step 2,
jump off both feet, lift your left
knee as high as you can, and
let your right foot leave the
ground completely.

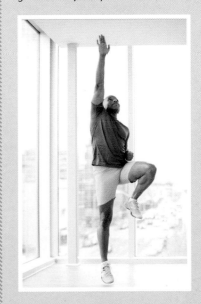

IMPROVES
■/// **Strength**
■/// **Stability**
■/// **Endurance**

WHAT YOU NEED
Dumbbells

Farmer's walk

A full shopping bag sometimes weighs as much as 9kg (20 pounds). Carrying heavy items like this requires coordination, stability, and strength, and performing this controlled forwards walk will prepare your body for weighted locomotion.

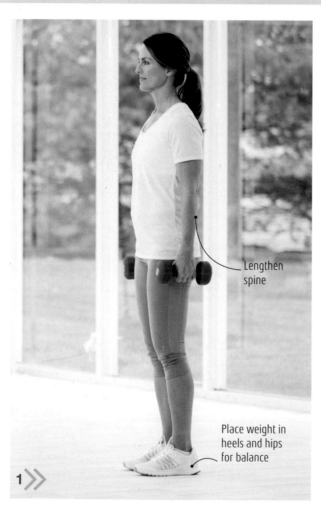

Lengthen spine

Place weight in heels and hips for balance

1 ⟩⟩

Stand with your feet shoulder-width apart. Hold a dumbbell in each hand, palms facing inwards, and let your arms hang at your sides. Engage your core and retract your shoulder blades.

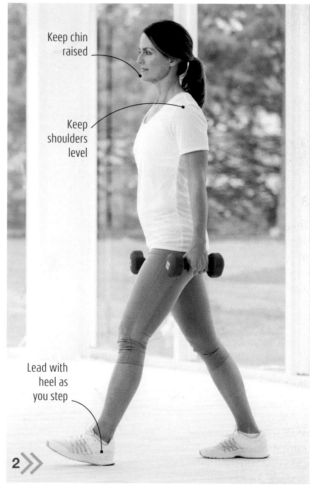

Keep chin raised

Keep shoulders level

Lead with heel as you step

2 ⟩⟩

Take a long step forwards with your left foot by engaging your hamstrings and glutes to pull your left heel forwards. Land with your heel first. Maintain a stable, upright posture.

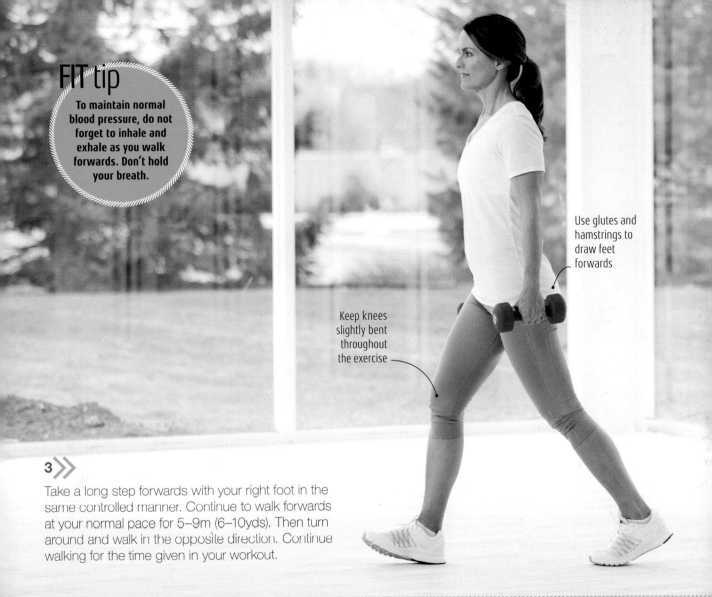

FIT tip

To maintain normal blood pressure, do not forget to inhale and exhale as you walk forwards. Don't hold your breath.

Use glutes and hamstrings to draw feet forwards

Keep knees slightly bent throughout the exercise

3 »

Take a long step forwards with your right foot in the same controlled manner. Continue to walk forwards at your normal pace for 5–9m (6–10yds). Then turn around and walk in the opposite direction. Continue walking for the time given in your workout.

MAKE IT easier

If it is difficult to maintain balance, don't use dumbbells. March in place by raising your knee straight up until your thigh is parallel to the ground then lowering it to the starting position. Repeat with the opposite leg.

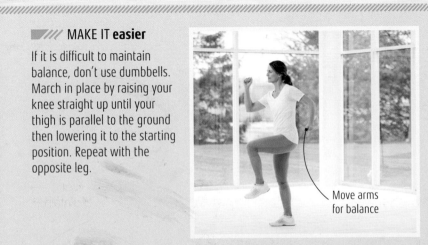

Move arms for balance

Skaters

Plyometric training, also known as jump training, involves rapidly stretching and contracting muscles to develop strength. Perform this quick plyometric drill to strengthen your legs and joints and improve your balance.

IMPROVES

▰/// Strength

▰/// Stability

▰/// Endurance

WHAT YOU NEED

No equipment needed

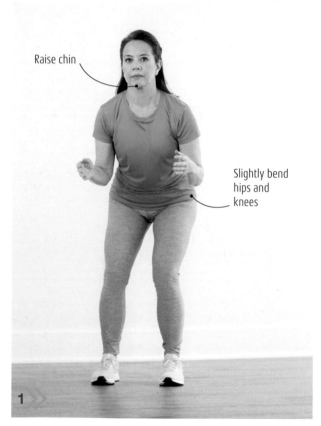

Raise chin

Slightly bend hips and knees

1

Stand with your feet shoulder-width apart. Bend your elbows to 90 degrees, position your forearms in front of you, and relax your hands. Slightly lean forwards, engage your core, and retract your shoulder blades.

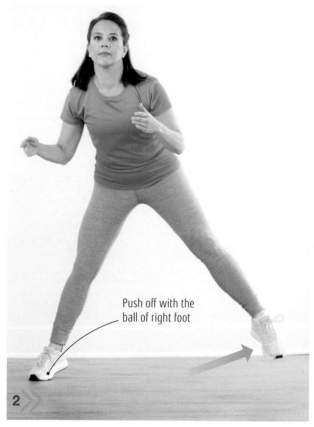

Push off with the ball of right foot

2

Push into the ground with your right foot, rising onto the ball of your foot, and extend your left leg out to the side to jump to your left. Keep your back lengthened and continue to lean slightly forwards.

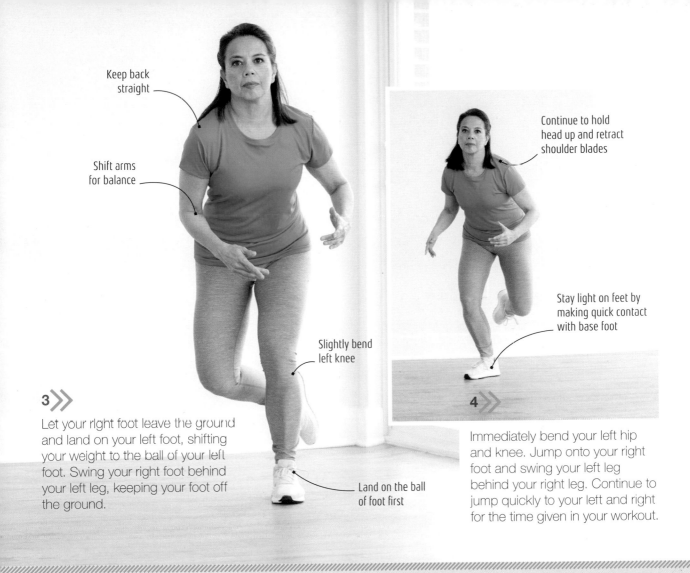

Keep back straight

Shift arms for balance

Slightly bend left knee

Continue to hold head up and retract shoulder blades

Stay light on feet by making quick contact with base foot

3 »

Let your right foot leave the ground and land on your left foot, shifting your weight to the ball of your left foot. Swing your right foot behind your left leg, keeping your foot off the ground.

Land on the ball of foot first

4 »

Immediately bend your left hip and knee. Jump onto your right foot and swing your left leg behind your right leg. Continue to jump quickly to your left and right for the time given in your workout.

▰/// MAKE IT **easier**

To lessen the impact on your joints, in step 2, step your left foot to the side rather than jumping. In step 3, pull your heel up towards your glutes rather than behind your base leg. Continue to step quickly to your left and right.

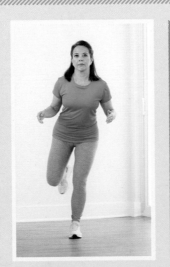

▰/// MAKE IT **harder**

To develop power in your lower body, in step 3, immediately upon landing on your left foot, squat down until your left thigh is parallel to the ground. Shift your arms for balance.

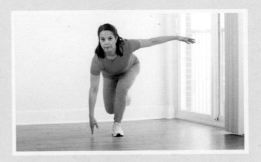

IMPROVES

▰/// **Strength**

▰/// **Stability**

▰/// **Mobility**

▰/// **Endurance**

WHAT YOU NEED

Step

Step-ups

A body with unhealthy knees is like a car with four flat tyres – you can still run, but you will not go far. Briskly perform this elevated stepping exercise to develop stability and strength in the muscles and connective tissues surrounding your knees so you can run more efficiently.

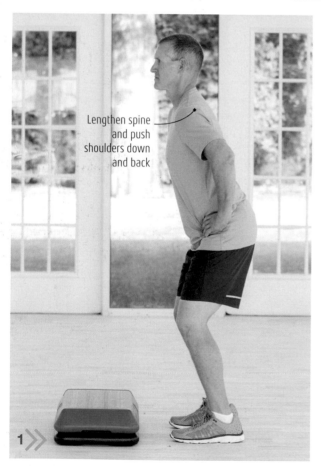

Lengthen spine and push shoulders down and back

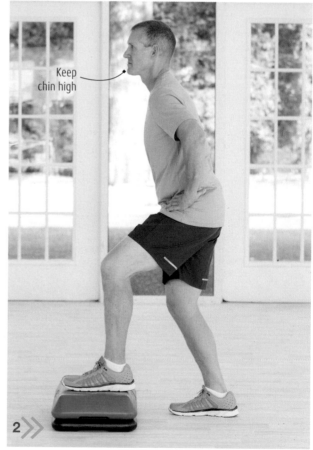

Keep chin high

1 >> Stand behind a step or stair with your feet shoulder-width apart and place your hands on your hips. Slightly lean forwards and bend your knees and hips. Engage your core and retract your shoulder blades.

2 >> Lift your left leg from the knee until your left foot is about 5cm (2in) above the step, then place your foot fully on the step, maintaining a shoulder-width distance between your feet.

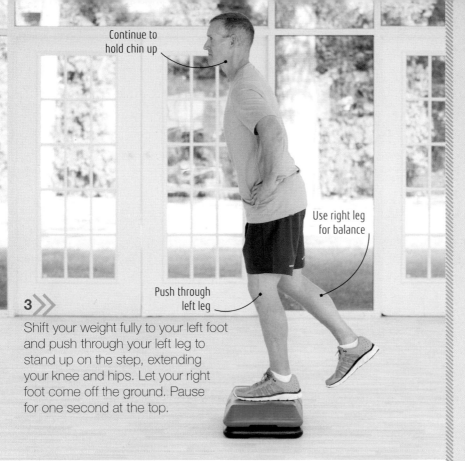

Continue to hold chin up

Use right leg for balance

Push through left leg

3 ▶▶

Shift your weight fully to your left foot and push through your left leg to stand up on the step, extending your knee and hips. Let your right foot come off the ground. Pause for one second at the top.

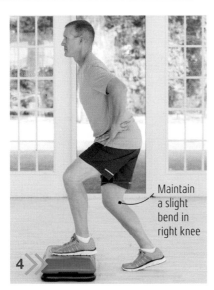

Maintain a slight bend in right knee

4 ▶▶

Lower your body back onto your right foot by bending your knees and hips. Shift your weight back to your right foot.

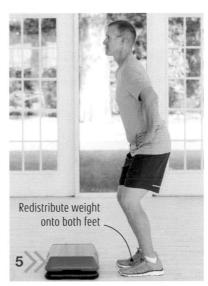

Redistribute weight onto both feet

5 ▶▶

Lift your left leg and return to the starting position. Alternate stepping with your left and right foot for the time given in your workout.

//// MAKE IT **easier**

If it is difficult to maintain balance, lightly rest your hand on a chair or rail for support.

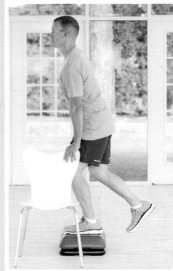

//// MAKE IT **harder**

To increase resistance to your legs, hold a dumbbell in each hand and let them hang at your sides throughout the exercise.

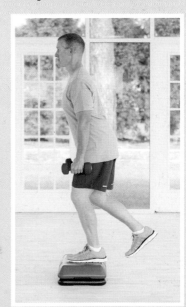

IMPROVES
▨//// Posture
▰//// Strength
▰//// Stability
▨//// Mobility
▰//// Endurance

WHAT YOU NEED
Dumbbells

Cross-country skiers

A strong, stable core enables the nervous system to engage your muscles better for functional movements. Your transverse abdominal, whose primary role is to stabilize your spine and pelvis, is the deepest abdominal muscle in your body. Use this fast-paced drill to strengthen this core muscle and protect your lower back.

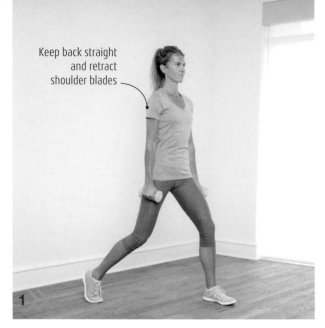

Keep back straight and retract shoulder blades

Hold a dumbbell in each hand and let your arms hang at your sides. Stand with your feet shoulder-width apart and step your right leg back into a staggered stance. Rise up onto the ball of your right foot and slightly bend your knees.

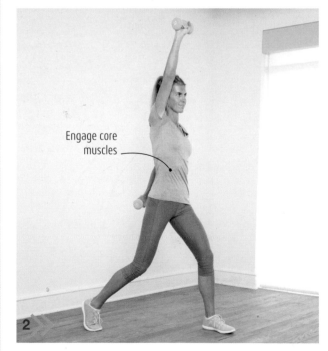

Engage core muscles

Swing your right arm forwards from the shoulder and lift until your upper arm is near your ear. Pull your left arm behind your body. Keep both arms straight as you move them.

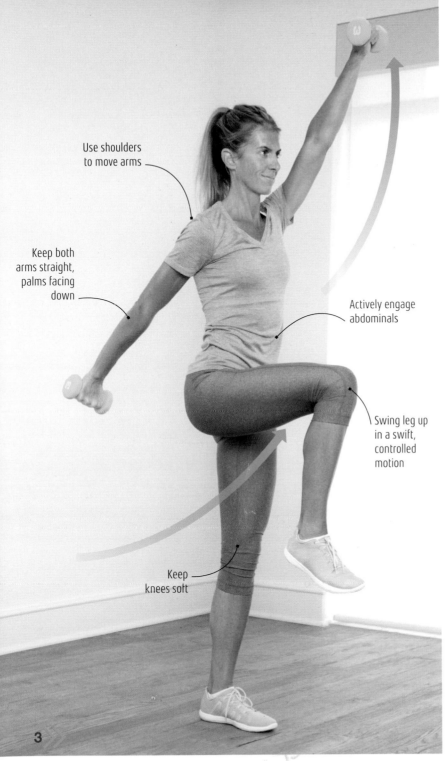

Use shoulders to move arms

Keep both arms straight, palms facing down

Actively engage abdominals

Swing leg up in a swift, controlled motion

Keep knees soft

3

Shift your weight to your left foot and use your core to raise your right knee until your thigh is parallel to the ground. Simultaneously swing your left arm up and forwards, and swing your right arm down and back.

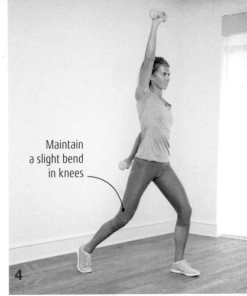

Maintain a slight bend in knees

4

In one swift motion, lower your right leg and swing your arms to reverse positions. Repeat the exercise for the time given in your workout. Spend half the time raising your right leg, then reverse your stance and raise your left leg.

//// MAKE IT **easier**

If it is difficult to maintain balance, do the exercise without dumbbells.

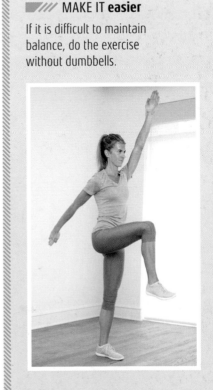

Faux skipping

Skipping is excellent for increasing the bone density of your legs. Since both legs absorb each jump, it's easier on the joints than running, while the weight-bearing impact keeps bones healthy and stable. Try this rope-free version.

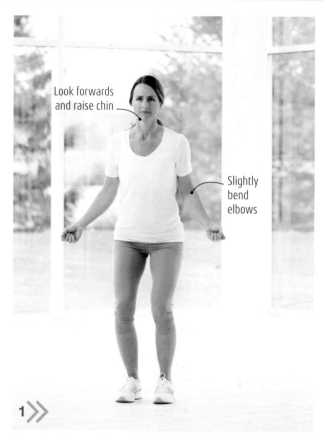

Look forwards and raise chin

Slightly bend elbows

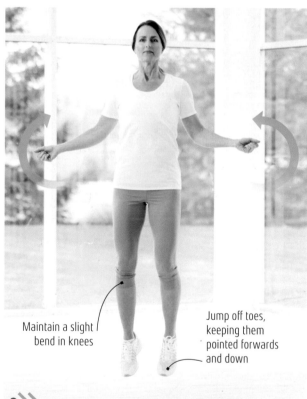

Maintain a slight bend in knees

Jump off toes, keeping them pointed forwards and down

1 ≫

Stand with your feet shoulder-width apart and slightly bend your knees. Hold your hands in loose fists, palms facing forwards, and bring them to waist height. Lengthen your torso and retract your shoulder blades.

2 ≫

Powerfully jump off the balls of your feet, 3–8cm (1–3in) into the air. Simultaneously draw a small, forwards circle with your wrists. Limit movement in your shoulders and elbows.

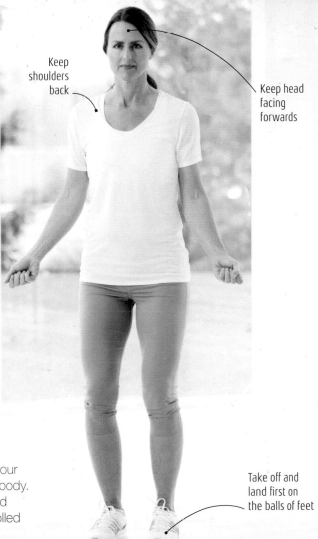

FIT tip

To get into the rhythm of skipping, try to keep your jumps as small as possible and maintain a consistent pace.

Keep shoulders back

Keep head facing forwards

3 »

Land softly on the balls of your feet and bend your knees to distribute the impact throughout your body. Quickly rebound back up into the next jump and wrist circle. Continue to jump with quick, controlled movements for the time given in your workout.

Take off and land first on the balls of feet

▰/// MAKE IT **easier**

To lessen impact, raise one foot off the ground at a time, alternating feet. Continue the sequence quickly with one wrist circle per step. Keep your heels off the ground.

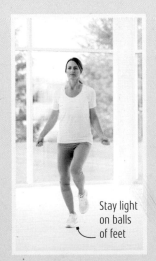

Stay light on balls of feet

▰/// MAKE IT **harder**

To improve reaction time, do the exercise with a skipping rope. Hold a handle in each hand and put the rope behind your heels. Jump and use your wrists to swing the rope behind you, over your head, and then under your feet.

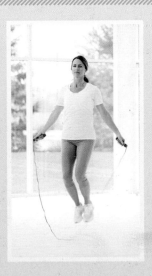

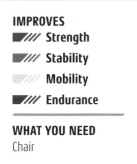

IMPROVES

▰/// **Strength**

▰/// **Stability**

/// **Mobility**

▰/// **Endurance**

WHAT YOU NEED
Chair

Chair mountain climber

This vigorous running exercise engages your whole body to improve your endurance and burn calories. Using only your bodyweight and a chair, the full-body movement increases the flexibility of your hips and strengthens your core and upper-body muscles.

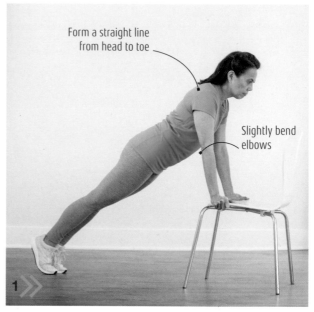

Form a straight line from head to toe

Slightly bend elbows

Stand facing the seat of a chair. Grip each side of the seat, step your feet back, and transfer your weight to your hands and the balls of your feet. Align your shoulders over your hands. Engage your core.

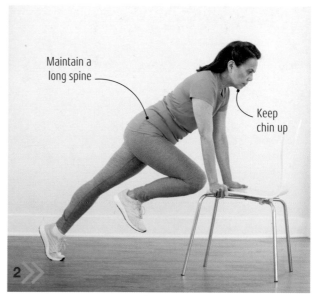

Maintain a long spine

Keep chin up

Push off the ball of your right foot and raise your right knee until your thigh is perpendicular to your left leg. Keep your core engaged and your shoulders square to the seat.

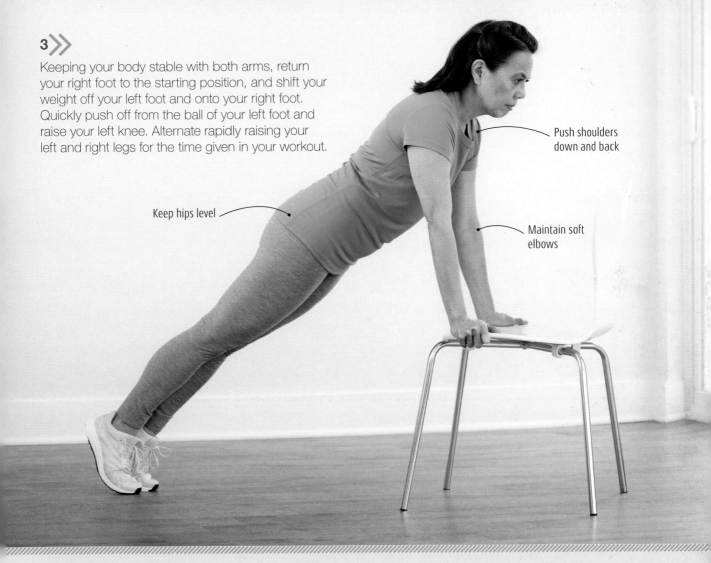

3 »

Keeping your body stable with both arms, return your right foot to the starting position, and shift your weight off your left foot and onto your right foot. Quickly push off from the ball of your left foot and raise your left knee. Alternate rapidly raising your left and right legs for the time given in your workout.

Push shoulders down and back

Keep hips level

Maintain soft elbows

▰/// MAKE IT easier

To reduce resistance to your core, place your hands on a wall at shoulder height and step your feet back until your body is at about a 45-degree angle to the ground. Do the exercise from this position.

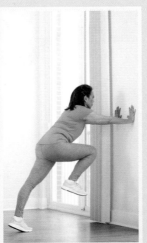

▰/// MAKE IT harder

To increase resistance to your core and upper body, do the exercise on the ground instead of with a chair.

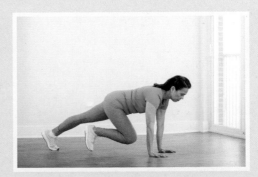

Switch jumps

Vigorous compound movements like this jumping exercise develop lower-body strength and power while improving your cardiovascular endurance. Use this dynamic drill to challenge your stability and make you more agile.

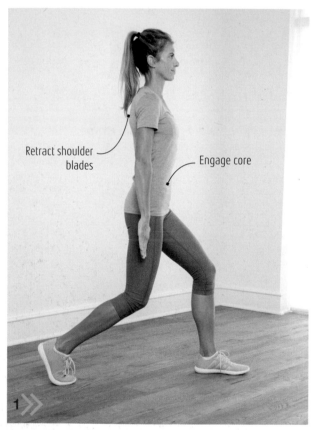

Retract shoulder blades

Engage core

1

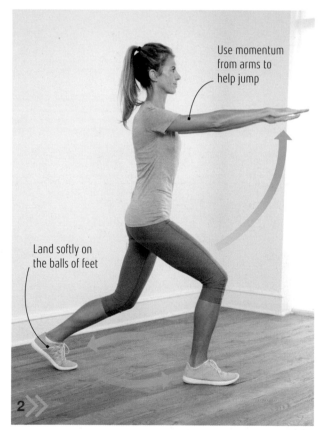

Use momentum from arms to help jump

Land softly on the balls of feet

2

Stand with your feet shoulder-width apart and straighten your arms at your sides with your palms facing behind you. Step your right leg back into a staggered stance and rise up onto the ball of your right foot. Slightly bend your knees.

Spring up off the balls of your feet to jump 2–5cm (1–2in) into the air, and switch your legs, bringing your right leg forwards and left leg backwards. At the same time, swing your arms straight up so they are parallel to the ground.

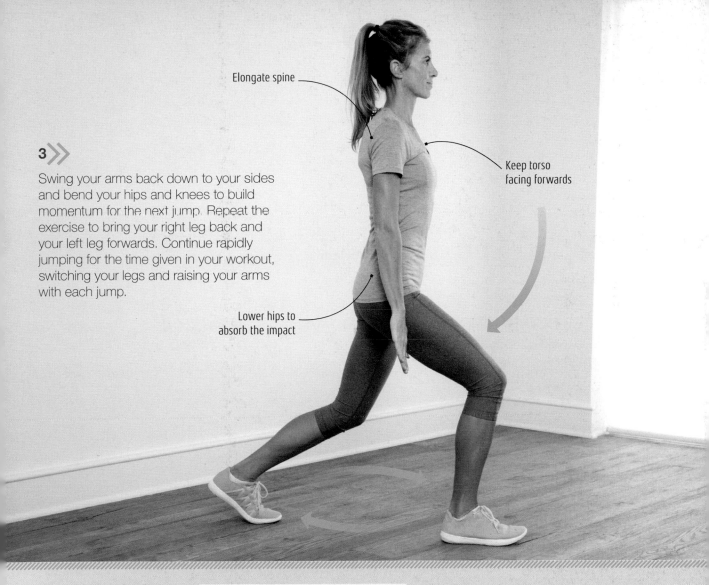

Elongate spine

Keep torso
facing forwards

3 »

Swing your arms back down to your sides
and bend your hips and knees to build
momentum for the next jump. Repeat the
exercise to bring your right leg back and
your left leg forwards. Continue rapidly
jumping for the time given in your workout,
switching your legs and raising your arms
with each jump.

Lower hips to
absorb the impact

//// **MAKE IT harder**

To strengthen your lower
body, between each jump,
drop your back knee into a
lunge until both knees are
bent to 90 degrees. Then
jump off the balls of your feet
and switch your legs.

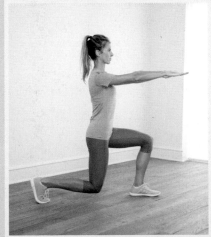

One-arm military press

This one-arm press teaches your body to transfer force from your core to your upper body. The controlled pushing movement challenges the stability of your entire body while strengthening the triceps and shoulders. By including this type of exercise in your regime, you'll be better able to stand tall throughout your day.

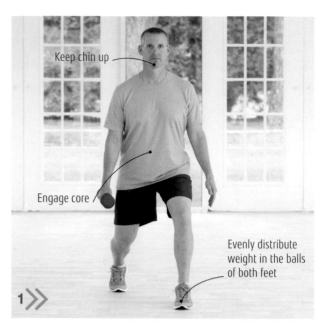

Keep chin up

Engage core

Evenly distribute weight in the balls of both feet

1 ≫

Hold a dumbbell in your right hand. Stand with your feet shoulder-width apart and step your right leg back into a staggered stance. Rise up onto the ball of your right foot. Slightly bend your knees.

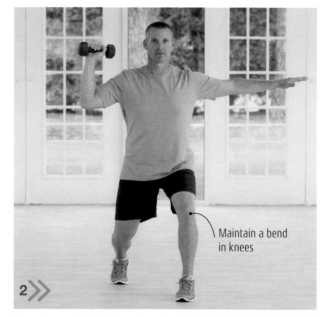

Maintain a bend in knees

2 ≫

Bend your right elbow to raise the dumbbell to chin height, palm facing forwards and forearm perpendicular to the ground. Extend your left arm out to your side with your palm facing the ground.

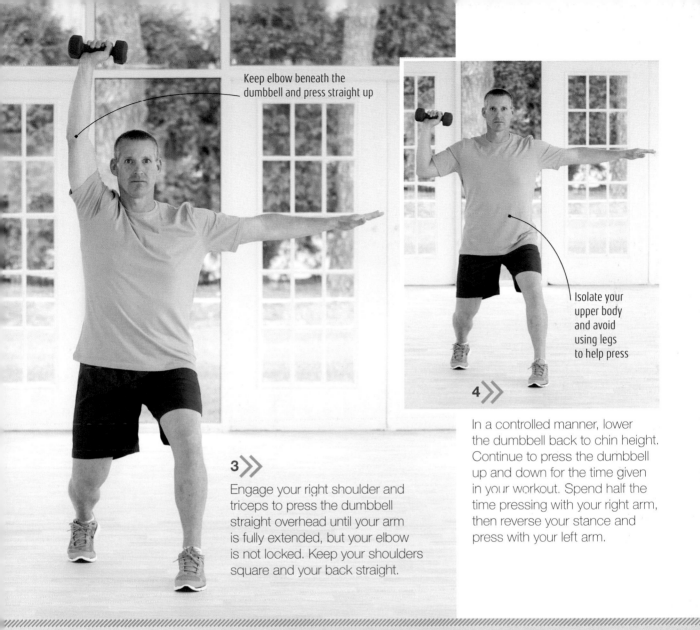

Keep elbow beneath the dumbbell and press straight up

Isolate your upper body and avoid using legs to help press

4 》》

In a controlled manner, lower the dumbbell back to chin height. Continue to press the dumbbell up and down for the time given in your workout. Spend half the time pressing with your right arm, then reverse your stance and press with your left arm.

3 》》

Engage your right shoulder and triceps to press the dumbbell straight overhead until your arm is fully extended, but your elbow is not locked. Keep your shoulders square and your back straight.

▰▰/// MAKE IT easier

If it is difficult to maintain balance, sit on the edge of a chair while performing the exercise.

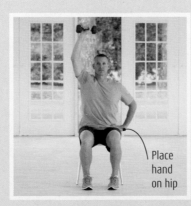

Place hand on hip

Chair dips

IMPROVES
▰/// **Strength**
/// Mobility
▰/// **Endurance**

WHAT YOU NEED
Chair

Many pushing activities, such as steering a pram or shopping trolley, require a strong upper body. Use this compound exercise to develop strength in your triceps, shoulders, chest, and back so you can perform these daily functions with ease.

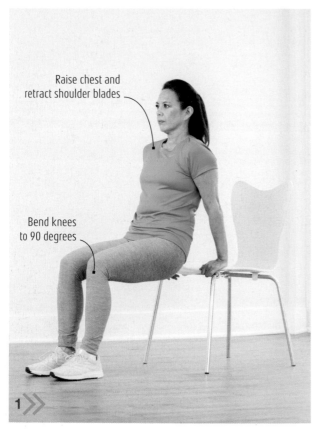

Raise chest and retract shoulder blades

Bend knees to 90 degrees

1 ⟫

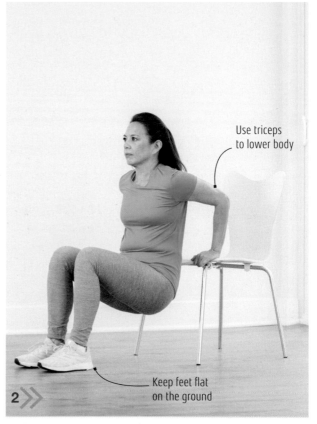

Use triceps to lower body

Keep feet flat on the ground

2 ⟫

Sit on a chair with your hands positioned shoulder-width apart and next to your hips on the edge of the chair. Extend your arms and press your body up onto the palms of your hands. Walk your feet out so your hips are suspended in front of the chair.

Engage your triceps, chest, and shoulders and bend your elbows to lower your hips and torso straight down. Lower your body until your elbows are bent to 90 degrees. Keep your chin raised and your chest upright.

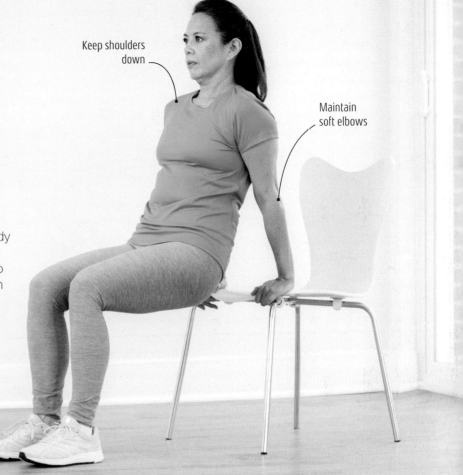

FIT tip

If you do not have a chair available, use any other sturdy object, such as a railing, low table, or the edge of a bathtub.

Keep shoulders down

Maintain soft elbows

3 »

Press your palms into the chair and extend your elbows to raise your body back to the starting position. Avoid using your legs to assist. Continue to repeat the exercise for the time given in your workout.

//// MAKE IT easier

To reduce resistance, do not walk your feet out in step 1 and keep your hips over the chair. In step 2, bend your elbows to lower your body back to a seated position.

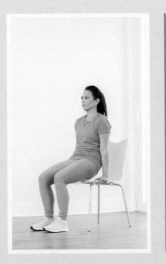

//// MAKE IT harder

To increase resistance, in step 1, walk your feet out until your legs are straight. Balance on your heels and keep your hips aligned under your torso.

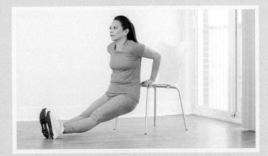

IMPROVES
/// **Posture**
/// **Strength**
/// **Stability**
/// **Mobility**
/// **Endurance**

WHAT YOU NEED
Countertop

Inclined push-ups

Few exercises are more efficient and effective than the push-up. This foundational movement, made easier on a raised surface, activates nearly every muscle in your body to improve posture, strengthen the upper body, develop core stability, and enhance shoulder mobility.

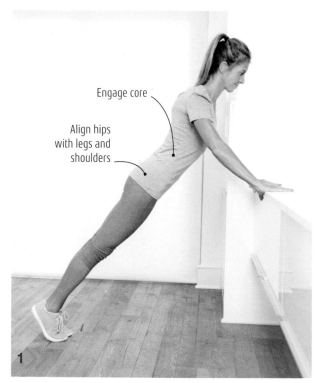

Engage core

Align hips with legs and shoulders

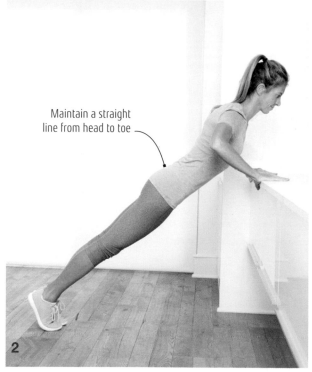

Maintain a straight line from head to toe

1 Stand facing a countertop, table, or other stable surface at about hip height. Place your hands shoulder-width apart on the edge of the surface. Step your feet back and transfer your weight to your hands.

2 In a controlled manner, bend your elbows and use your triceps, chest, and shoulders to lower your body until your elbows are bent to 90 degrees. Maintain a flat back and keep your core tight.

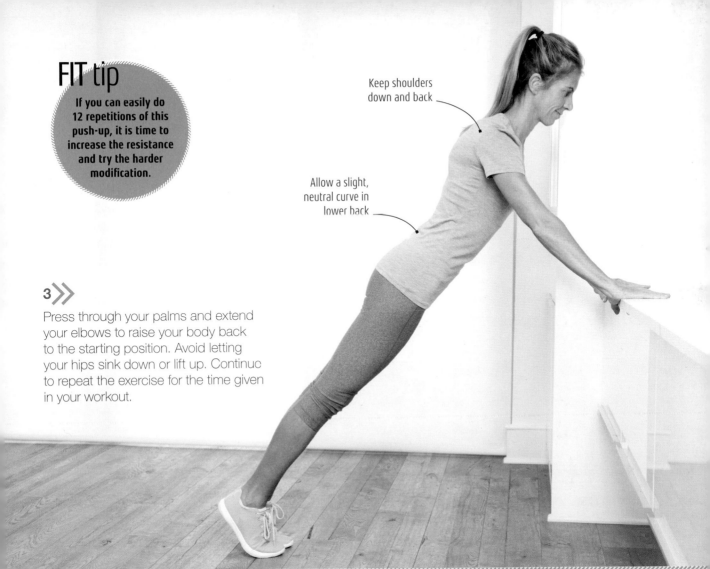

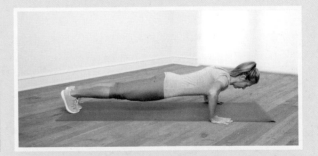

FIT tip

If you can easily do 12 repetitions of this push-up, it is time to increase the resistance and try the harder modification.

Keep shoulders down and back

Allow a slight, neutral curve in lower back

3 »

Press through your palms and extend your elbows to raise your body back to the starting position. Avoid letting your hips sink down or lift up. Continue to repeat the exercise for the time given in your workout.

▰/// MAKE IT easier

To reduce resistance to your upper body, place your hands on a wall at shoulder height and step your feet back until your body is at a 45-degree angle to the ground. Do the push-up from this position.

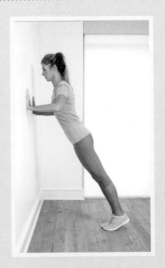

▰/// MAKE IT harder

To increase resistance to your core and upper body, do the exercise on the ground. Align your shoulders directly over your hands, fingers pointing forwards.

IMPROVES

//// **Stability**

//// **Mobility**

//// **Endurance**

WHAT YOU NEED
Dumbbells

Curl and shoulder press and reach

Reaching overhead requires coordination and stability in your legs, core, and upper body. Perform this exercise so you are more prepared the next time you need to place an object on a high shelf or cupboard.

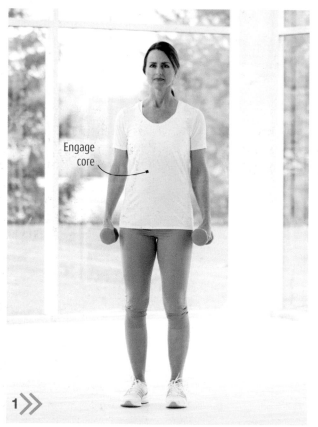

Engage core

1 »

Stand with your feet shoulder-width apart. Hold a dumbbell in each hand and let your arms hang at your sides. Slightly bend your knees. Lengthen your torso and retract your shoulder blades.

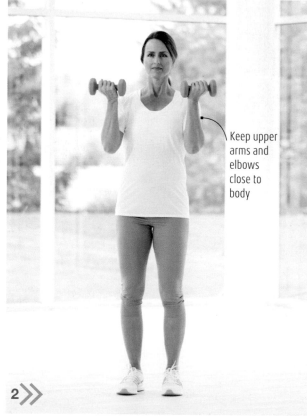

Keep upper arms and elbows close to body

2 »

In a controlled manner, with your palms facing forwards, engage your biceps to curl the dumbbells to shoulder height. Raise them through your elbows, which act as hinges.

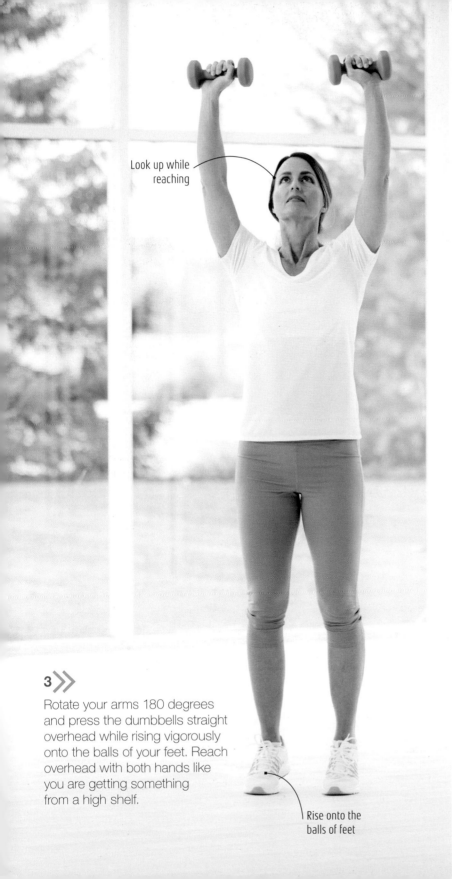

Look up while reaching

Rise onto the balls of feet

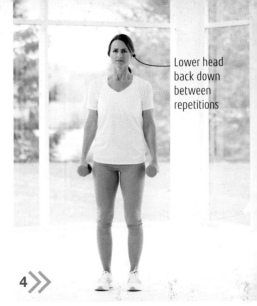

Lower head back down between repetitions

4 »

Lower your heels and return the dumbbells to the curl position, then back to the starting position. Continue to repeat the exercise for the time given in your workout.

3 »

Rotate your arms 180 degrees and press the dumbbells straight overhead while rising vigorously onto the balls of your feet. Reach overhead with both hands like you are getting something from a high shelf.

//// **MAKE IT easier**

To decrease resistance, use an exercise ball rather than dumbbells. Hold it down in front of you, curl it to shoulder height, then press and reach overhead.

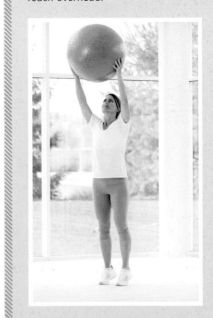

IMPROVES

/// **Posture**

/// **Mobility**

WHAT YOU NEED
No equipment needed

Chest opener

Many daily activities require you to have your arms in front of you – lifting objects, holding a steering wheel, using your phone, or typing on a keyboard. Holding these positions for prolonged periods of time can result in tight shoulders and chest muscles. Use this chest stretch to loosen your upper-body muscles and improve your flexibility and posture.

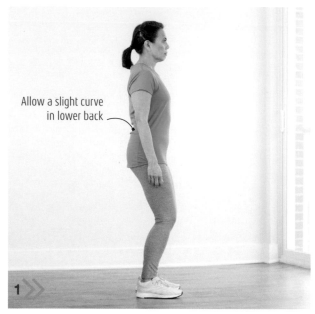

Allow a slight curve in lower back

Stand with your feet shoulder-width apart and let your arms hang at your sides. Lengthen your torso and retract your shoulder blades. Slightly bend your knees.

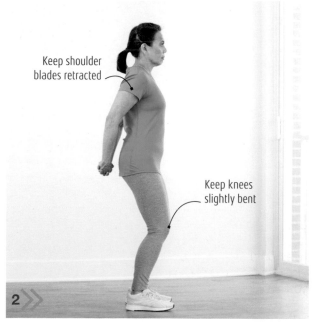

Keep shoulder blades retracted

Keep knees slightly bent

Bring your hands behind your back and interlock your fingers. Keep your head raised and shoulders back.

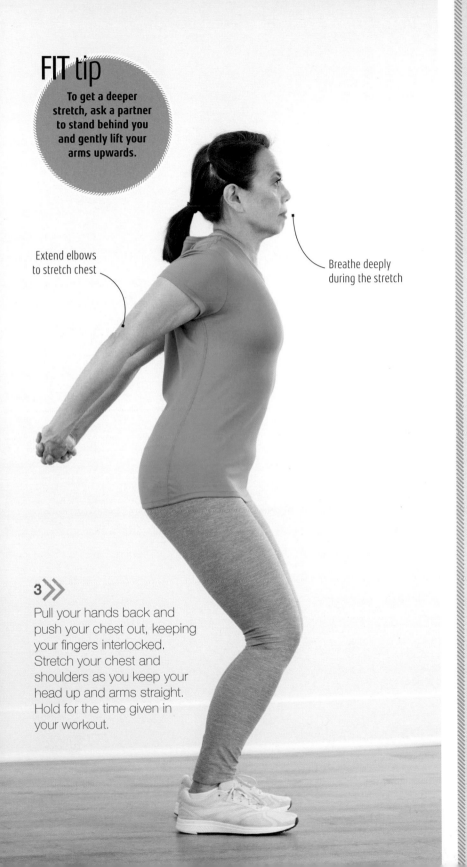

FIT tip

To get a deeper stretch, ask a partner to stand behind you and gently lift your arms upwards.

Extend elbows to stretch chest

Breathe deeply during the stretch

3 ≫

Pull your hands back and push your chest out, keeping your fingers interlocked. Stretch your chest and shoulders as you keep your head up and arms straight. Hold for the time given in your workout.

▰/// MAKE IT **easier**

If it is difficult to clasp your hands behind you, extend one arm behind you, parallel to the ground, and grab a stable surface. Turn your body away from your arm to open your chest. Repeat with the other arm.

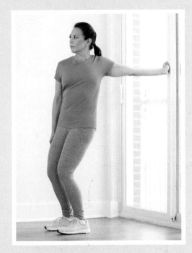

▰/// MAKE IT **harder**

To increase the intensity of the stretch, bend over at your waist, using your hips as a hinge, and pull your arms forwards.

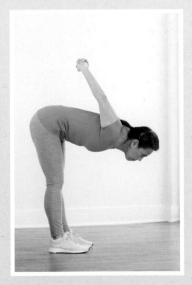

IMPROVES
/// Posture
/// Strength
/// Stability
/// Mobility
/// Endurance

WHAT YOU NEED
Dumbbells

Push press

Transferring weight from your lower to upper body requires immense central nervous system coordination. Use this dynamic overhead strength exercise to enhance your motor skills and improve your ability for actions such as lifting a box or suitcase overhead.

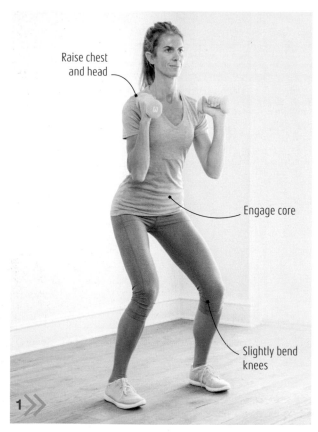

Raise chest and head

Engage core

Slightly bend knees

1 »

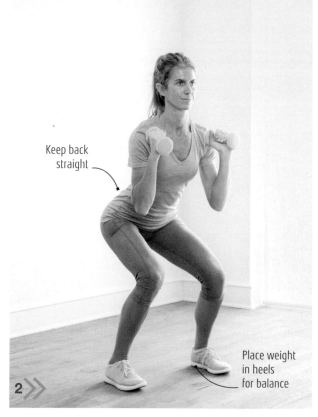

Keep back straight

Place weight in heels for balance

2 »

Stand with your feet slightly wider than shoulder-width apart and hold a dumbbell in each hand. Hold the dumbbells at shoulder height, palms facing each other, and keep your elbows close to your body.

Push your glutes back and bend at your hips and knees. Squat until your knees are bent to 45 degrees. Face your knees forwards and keep your elbows close to your body.

Keep elbows soft

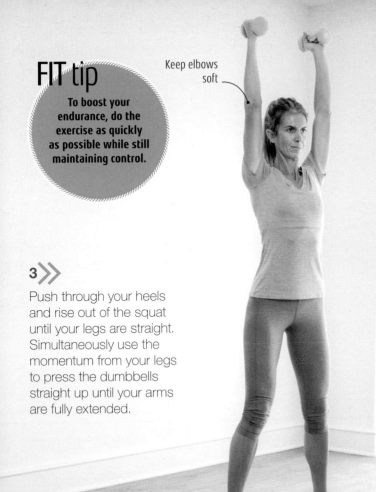

FIT tip

To boost your endurance, do the exercise as quickly as possible while still maintaining control.

3 »

Push through your heels and rise out of the squat until your legs are straight. Simultaneously use the momentum from your legs to press the dumbbells straight up until your arms are fully extended.

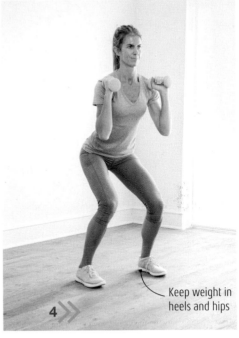

Keep weight in heels and hips

4 »

Lower the dumbbells back to your shoulders while bending your knees and hips to enter into the next squat. Continue to repeat the exercise for the time given in your workout.

//// MAKE IT **easier**

If it is difficult to maintain balance, sit on the edge of a chair while performing the exercise.

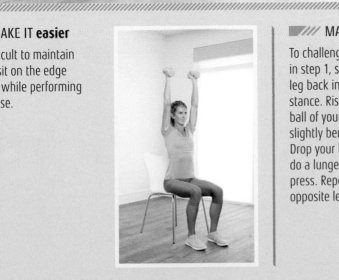

//// MAKE IT **harder**

To challenge your stability, in step 1, step your right leg back into a staggered stance. Rise up onto the ball of your right foot and slightly bend your knees. Drop your back knee and do a lunge between each press. Repeat with the opposite leg.

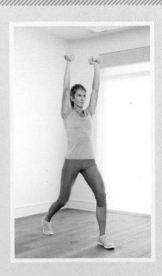

IMPROVES

▰//// **Posture**

▰//// **Strength**

▰//// **Stability**

▰//// **Endurance**

WHAT YOU NEED
Dumbbell

One-arm chest press

This balance exercise works one arm at a time, forcing your body to recruit your core muscles to keep your body stable and prevent you from tilting to the side. The controlled, unilateral movement is crucial for improving your core stability and correcting upper-body imbalances.

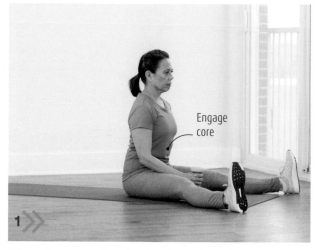

Engage core

Sit on the ground and extend your legs into a narrow v-shape. Firmly hold a dumbbell with your right hand and rest it between your legs. Rest your left hand on the ground for balance.

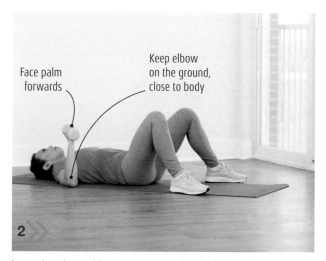

Face palm forwards

Keep elbow on the ground, close to body

Lean back and lay your upper body flat on the ground. Bend your knees and plant your feet slightly wider than hip-width apart. Rest your right upper arm on the ground and raise your forearm. Extend your left arm out to your side, palm facing down.

3 »

In a controlled manner, engage your chest, triceps, and shoulder to press the dumbbell straight up, fully extending your right arm. Keep the dumbbell aligned directly over your elbow. Avoid arching your lower back by drawing your belly button into the ground.

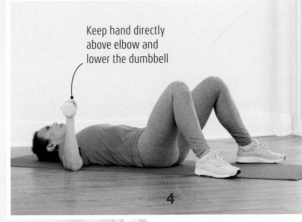

Keep hand directly above elbow and lower the dumbbell

4

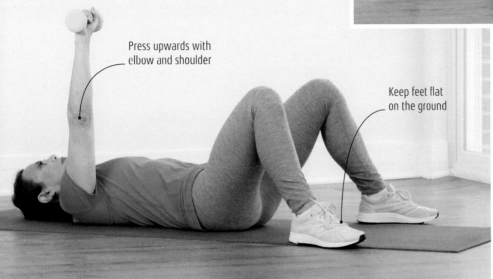

Press upwards with elbow and shoulder

Keep feet flat on the ground

Lower the dumbbell in a controlled manner by bending your right elbow until your upper arm is flat on the ground. Repeat the press for the time given in your workout. Spend half the time pressing with your right arm, then swap to your left arm.

▰/// MAKE IT **easier**

If it is difficult to maintain balance, hold a dumbbell in each hand and press both dumbbells up at the same time. Keep the dumbbells aligned directly over your elbows.

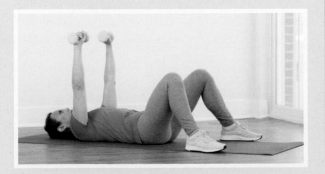

▰/// MAKE IT **harder**

To strengthen your glutes and hamstrings, drive your heels into the ground and lift your hips. Hold the position while you press and lower the dumbbell.

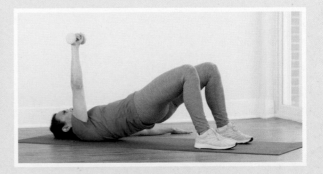

One-leg arm raise

Balance is essential for safely performing most activities, such as standing on one leg without falling over or maintaining control while walking. Do this controlled, one-legged drill to improve your stability.

IMPROVES
/// Posture
/// Strength
/// Stability

WHAT YOU NEED
Dumbbell

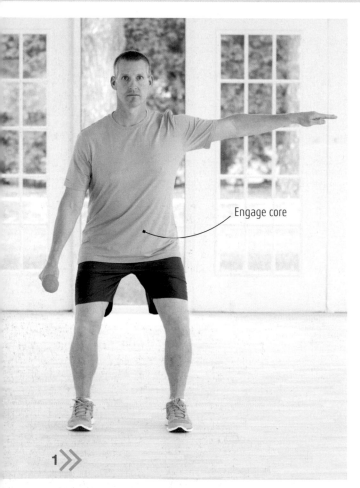

Engage core

1 »

Stand with your feet shoulder-width apart and slightly bend your knees. Hold a dumbbell in your right hand and let your arm hang at your side. Extend your left arm straight out to your side at shoulder height.

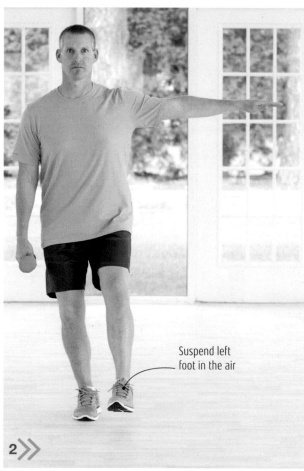

Suspend left foot in the air

2 »

Raise your left knee until your foot is about 8cm (3in) off the ground, and transfer your weight to your right heel. Maintain a slight bend in both knees and keep your core engaged.

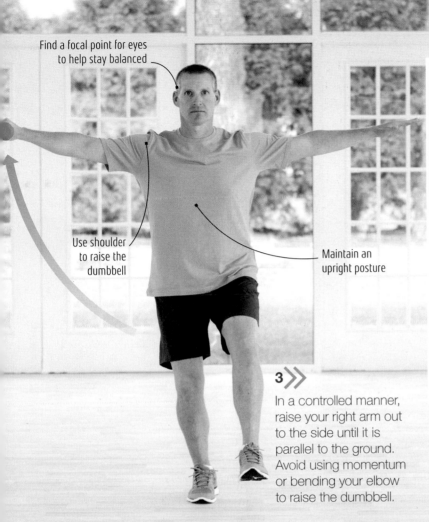

Find a focal point for eyes to help stay balanced

Use shoulder to raise the dumbbell

Maintain an upright posture

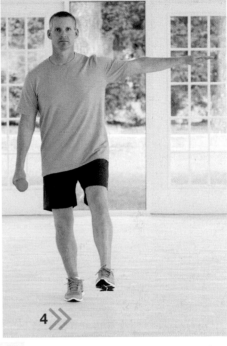

3 »

In a controlled manner, raise your right arm out to the side until it is parallel to the ground. Avoid using momentum or bending your elbow to raise the dumbbell.

4 »

Return the dumbbell to your side in a controlled manner. Keep your left foot raised and spend half the given time working your right arm. Then swap leg positions and repeat with the opposite arm.

//// **MAKE IT easier**

If it is difficult to balance, lightly rest your hand on a chair or wall for support, but avoid leaning into it or relying on it too much.

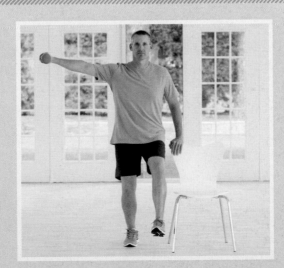

IMPROVES
/// Posture
/// **Strength**
/// **Stability**
/// Mobility
/// **Endurance**

WHAT YOU NEED
Wall

Jumping wall push-ups

Add speed and explosive power to an inclined push-up by pushing off the wall between each repetition. Jumping exercises like this one develop the nervous system and improve your coordination, motor skills, and balance. The increased upper-body power generated by this exercise is especially beneficial for golfers, tennis players, and swimmers.

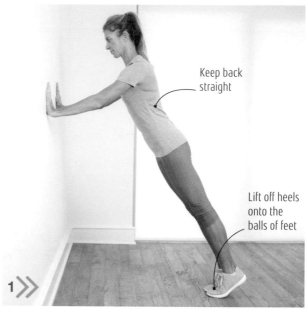

Keep back straight

Lift off heels onto the balls of feet

1 »

Place your hands on a wall keeping them shoulder-width apart and at chest height. Step your feet back until your body is about 45 degrees to the ground. Shift your weight to your hands and rise onto the balls of your feet.

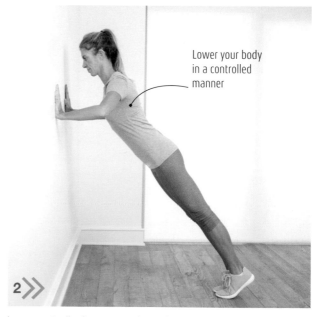

Lower your body in a controlled manner

2 »

In a controlled manner, bend your elbows and use your triceps, chest, and shoulders to lower your body until your elbows are bent to about 90 degrees. Keep your core engaged and your back straight.

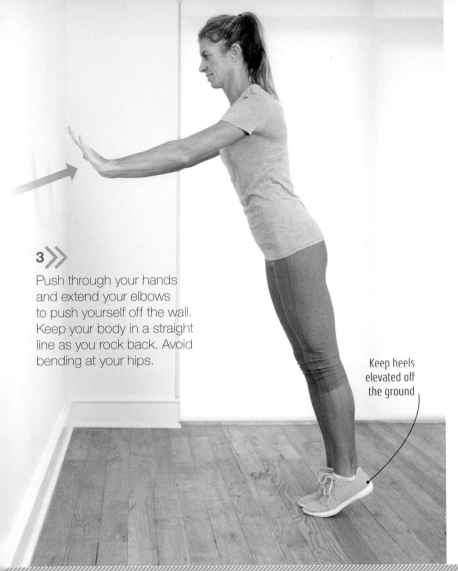

3 »

Push through your hands and extend your elbows to push yourself off the wall. Keep your body in a straight line as you rock back. Avoid bending at your hips.

Keep heels elevated off the ground

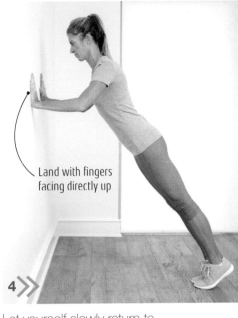

Land with fingers facing directly up

4 »

Let yourself slowly return to the wall. Catch yourself with your hands and bend your elbows to absorb the impact. Load your arms, chest, and shoulders for the next push-up, and repeat for the time given in your workout.

///// MAKE IT **easier**

To reduce the resistance to your upper body, stand closer to the wall. Step your feet back until your body is at about a 60-degree angle to the ground, and do the exercise from this position.

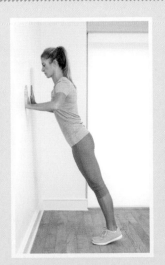

///// MAKE IT **harder**

To increase resistance to your core and upper body, do the exercise on the ground. Put your knees on the ground and lower your hips until your body is angled at about 45 degrees.

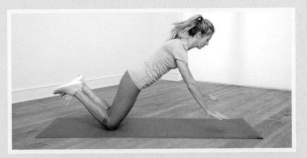

Gunslinger

IMPROVES
//// **Posture**
//// **Strength**
//// **Stability**

WHAT YOU NEED
Dumbbells

Your core connects your upper and lower body, but a weak connection can lead to poor balance. This weighted pushing exercise strengthens your core and enhances your body's head-to-toe coordination.

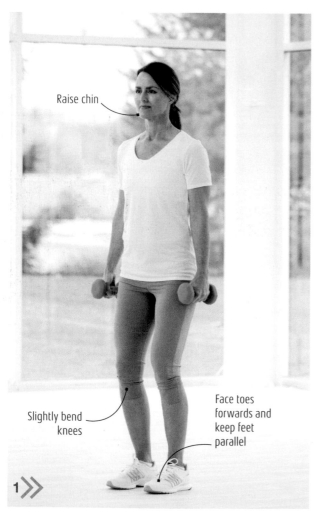

Raise chin

Slightly bend knees

Face toes forwards and keep feet parallel

1 》

Stand with your feet shoulder-width apart. Hold a dumbbell in each hand, palms facing inwards, and let your arms hang at your sides. Engage your core and retract your shoulder blades.

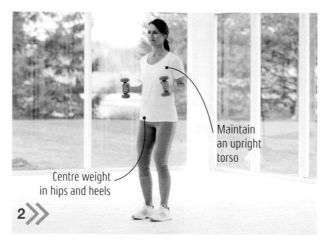

Maintain an upright torso

Centre weight in hips and heels

2 》

In a controlled manner, engage your biceps and forearms to curl the dumbbells until your forearms are parallel to the ground.

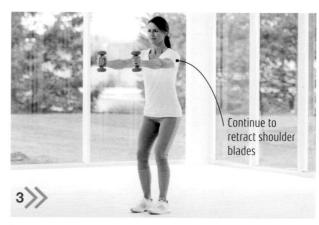

Continue to retract shoulder blades

3 》

In the same controlled manner, engage your chest and shoulders to push the dumbbells straight out until your arms are fully extended in front of you and parallel to the ground.

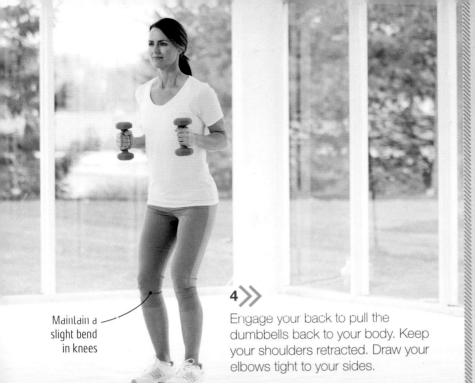

Maintain a slight bend in knees

4 »
Engage your back to pull the dumbbells back to your body. Keep your shoulders retracted. Draw your elbows tight to your sides.

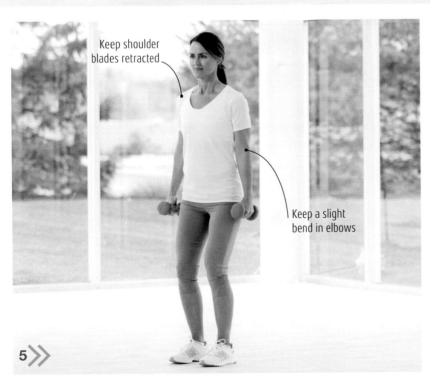

Keep shoulder blades retracted

Keep a slight bend in elbows

5 »
In a controlled manner, return the dumbbells to the starting position, and avoid hunching forwards. Repeat the sequence for the time given in your workout.

MAKE IT **easier**
To decrease the load on your lower back, sit on the edge of a chair while performing the exercise.

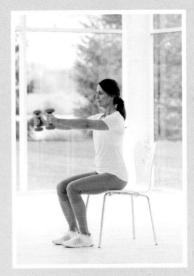

MAKE IT **harder**
To improve your balance, do the exercise from a staggered stance. In step 1, step your left leg back and rise up onto the ball of your left foot. Repeat in the opposite stance.

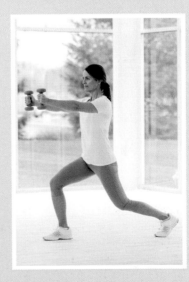

IMPROVES

▰/// **Strength**

▰/// **Stability**

/// **Mobility**

▰/// **Endurance**

WHAT YOU NEED
Dumbbell

Shot-put press

You do not have to be an Olympic athlete to benefit from increased rotational power and stability. This swift and controlled throwing exercise improves your coordination for sports like golf and tennis.

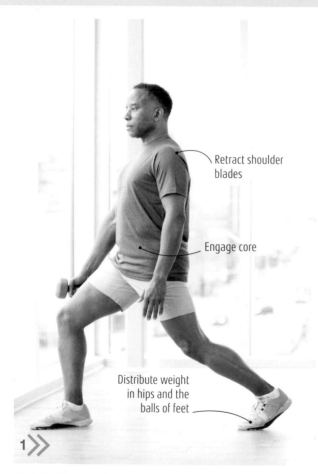

Retract shoulder blades

Engage core

Distribute weight in hips and the balls of feet

1 》》

Stand with your feet shoulder-width apart. Hold a dumbbell in your right hand and let your arms hang at your sides. Step your left leg back into a staggered stance and rise up onto the ball of your left foot.

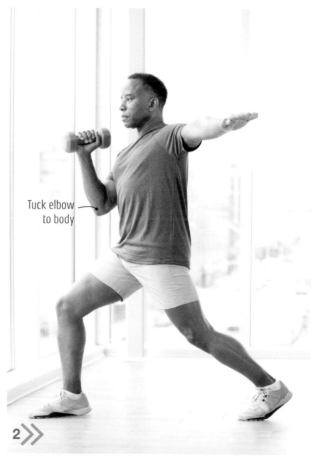

Tuck elbow to body

2 》》

Bend your right elbow to raise the dumbbell near your chin, palm facing inwards. Extend your left arm out to your side at a right angle to your body, palm facing the ground. Keep your core engaged.

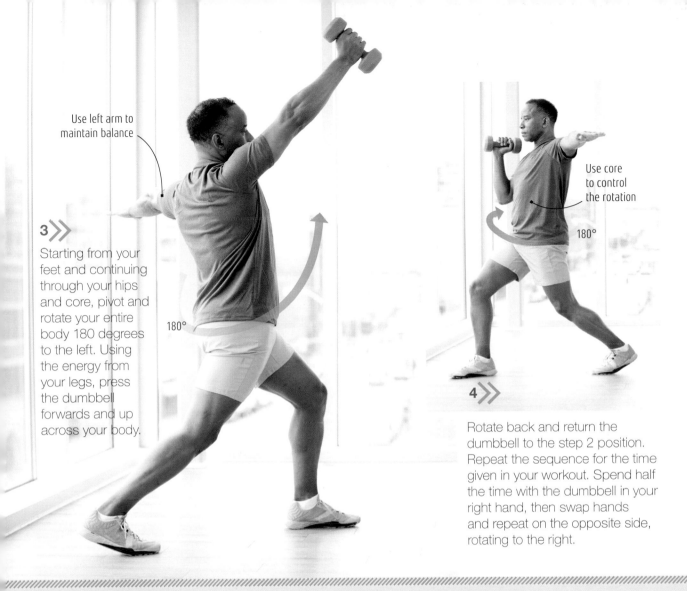

Use left arm to maintain balance

3 »

Starting from your feet and continuing through your hips and core, pivot and rotate your entire body 180 degrees to the left. Using the energy from your legs, press the dumbbell forwards and up across your body.

180°

Use core to control the rotation

180°

4 »

Rotate back and return the dumbbell to the step 2 position. Repeat the sequence for the time given in your workout. Spend half the time with the dumbbell in your right hand, then swap hands and repeat on the opposite side, rotating to the right.

▰/// MAKE IT **easier**

If it is difficult to maintain balance, do the exercise without a dumbbell. Hold your hand in a fist.

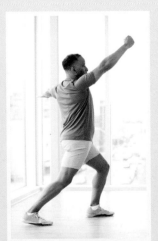

▰/// MAKE IT **harder**

To strengthen your legs, drop your back knee into a lunge before rotating in step 3. Rise back up into the staggered stance as you begin to rotate.

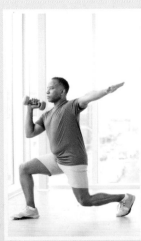

IMPROVES

/// Posture
/// Strength
/// Stability
/// Endurance

WHAT YOU NEED
Dumbbell

Suitcase row

Pulling with one arm at a time requires a strong and stable core. Use this quick and controlled unilateral movement to build back strength and improve stability for everyday activities such as weeding and lifting luggage.

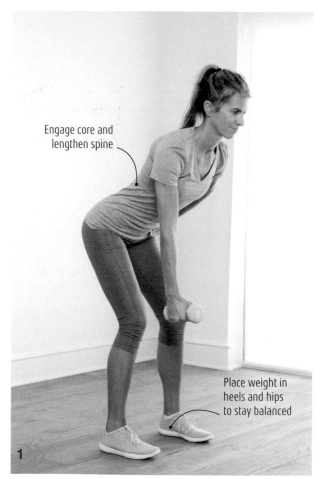

Engage core and lengthen spine

Place weight in heels and hips to stay balanced

1

Stand with your feet shoulder-width apart and bend over from the hips. Hold a dumbbell in your right hand and let your arm hang straight down. Put your left hand on your hip. Retract your shoulder blades.

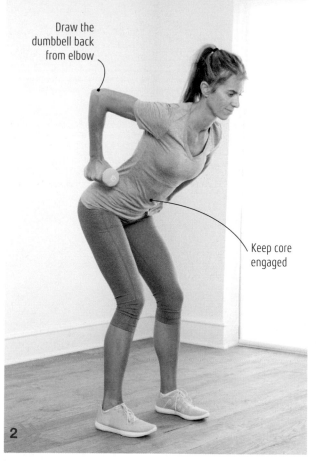

Draw the dumbbell back from elbow

Keep core engaged

2

Pull the dumbbell up and back from your elbow. Keep your shoulders square and your elbow tight to your body as you row. Contract your back at the top of the movement.

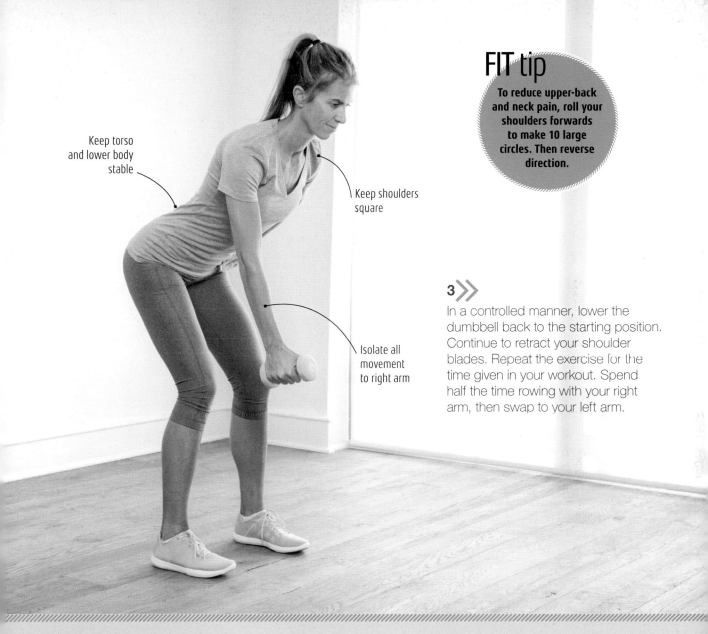

Keep torso
and lower body
stable

Keep shoulders
square

Isolate all
movement
to right arm

FIT tip

To reduce upper-back
and neck pain, roll your
shoulders forwards
to make 10 large
circles. Then reverse
direction.

3 »

In a controlled manner, lower the
dumbbell back to the starting position.
Continue to retract your shoulder
blades. Repeat the exercise for the
time given in your workout. Spend
half the time rowing with your right
arm, then swap to your left arm.

///// MAKE IT **easier**

If it is difficult to maintain
balance, sit on the edge of
a chair and bend forwards
while performing the exercise.

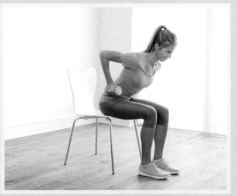

Lawn mower row

Twisting and pulling to start a lawn mower is the type of compound movement life often demands. This quick and controlled exercise improves the rotational strength and total-body coordination needed for this kind of pulling activity.

IMPROVES
▰/// **Strength**
▰/// **Stability**
/// Mobility
▰/// **Endurance**

WHAT YOU NEED
Dumbbell

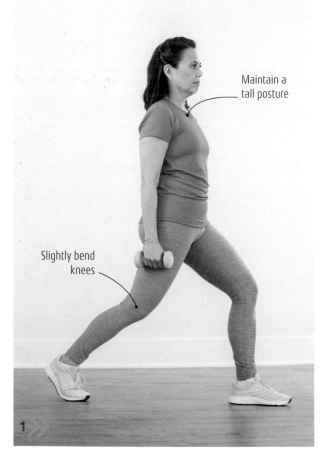

Maintain a tall posture

Slightly bend knees

1

Stand with your feet shoulder-width apart. Hold a dumbbell in your right hand, and let your arms hang at your sides. Step your right leg back into a staggered stance and rise up onto the ball of your right foot.

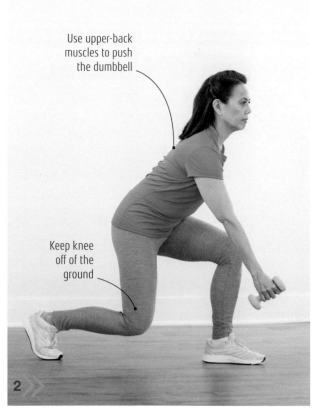

Use upper-back muscles to push the dumbbell

Keep knee off of the ground

2

Drop your right knee down until both knees are bent to 90 degrees. Simultaneously push the dumbbell forwards, towards your left toes, until your arm is fully extended. Centre your weight in both feet and hips.

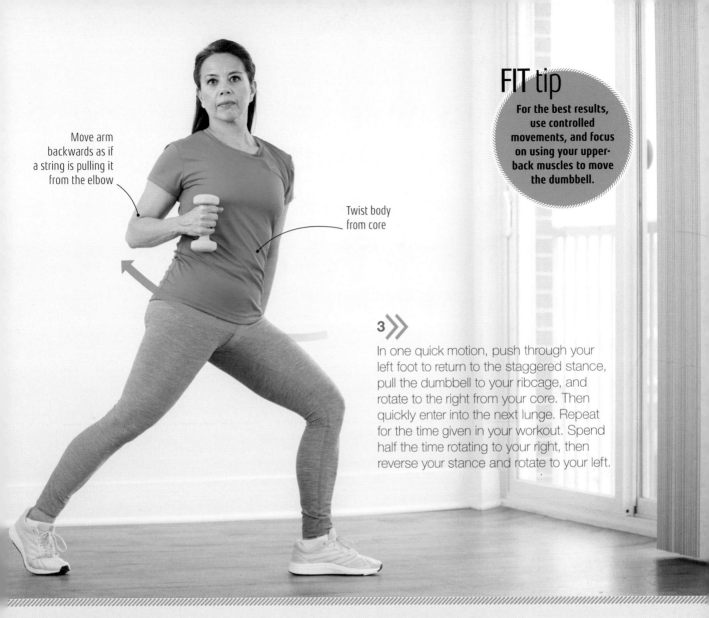

Move arm backwards as if a string is pulling it from the elbow

Twist body from core

FIT tip

For the best results, use controlled movements, and focus on using your upper-back muscles to move the dumbbell.

3 »

In one quick motion, push through your left foot to return to the staggered stance, pull the dumbbell to your ribcage, and rotate to the right from your core. Then quickly enter into the next lunge. Repeat for the time given in your workout. Spend half the time rotating to your right, then reverse your stance and rotate to your left.

//// MAKE IT **easier**

To decrease the load on your legs, in step 1, keep your feet in a neutral stance. In step 2, rather than lunging, sit your hips back into a squat.

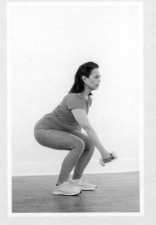

//// MAKE IT **harder**

To intensify the full-body coordination required, in step 1, step your left leg forwards rather than stepping your right foot back. In step 2, drop into a lunge as you reach forwards. In step 3, return your legs to the starting position by stepping your left leg back. Repeat on the opposite side.

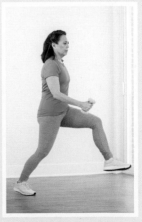

Staggered reverse fly

The human body is built to stand and move, so if you sit for many hours a day, it can lead to poor posture. Perform this quick upper-back exercise to improve your spinal alignment and strengthen your back.

IMPROVES
/// Posture
/// Strength
/// Stability
/// Mobility

WHAT YOU NEED
Dumbbells

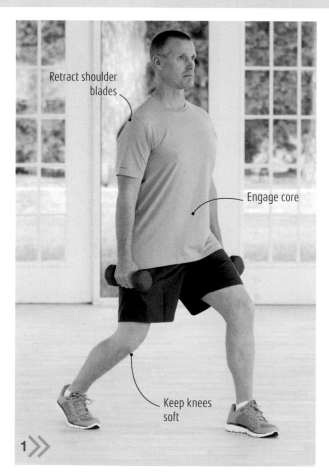

Retract shoulder blades

Engage core

Keep knees soft

1 ⟫

Hold a dumbbell in each hand. Stand with your feet shoulder-width apart and step your right leg back into a staggered stance. Rise up onto the ball of your right foot. Slightly bend your knees.

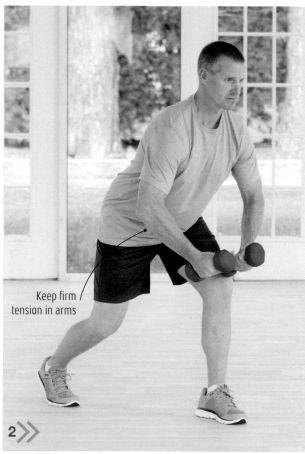

Keep firm tension in arms

2 ⟫

Bend over to 45 degrees from the hips and bring the dumbbells together. Slightly bend your elbows as if you are wrapping your arms around a tree trunk. Keep your back flat and your head raised.

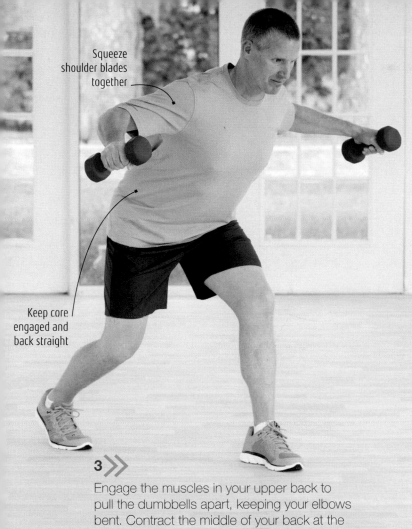

Squeeze
shoulder blades
together

Keep core
engaged and
back straight

3 »
Engage the muscles in your upper back to
pull the dumbbells apart, keeping your elbows
bent. Contract the middle of your back at the
top of the movement.

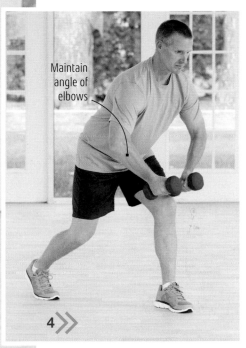

Maintain
angle of
elbows

4 »

Using your back muscles, return
the dumbbells to the starting
position. Repeat the exercise in
a quick, controlled manner for the
time given in your workout. Swap
your stance halfway through.

///// MAKE IT **easier**

If it is difficult to maintain
balance, sit on the edge of
a chair and lean forwards
at the hips while performing
the exercise.

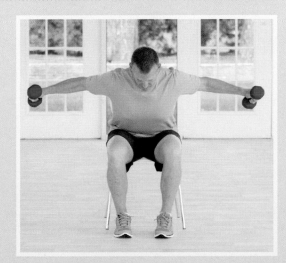

IMPROVES

/// Posture

/// Strength

/// Stability

/// Mobility

/// Endurance

WHAT YOU NEED
Dumbbells

Arm pullovers

Lack of shoulder mobility is one of the most common causes of upper-body injury. The rapid pulling motion in this exercise will help you to prevent injuries, improve mobility, and strengthen your shoulders and upper back for more functional movement.

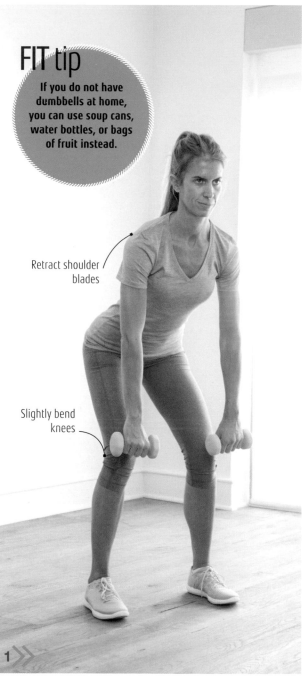

FIT tip
If you do not have dumbbells at home, you can use soup cans, water bottles, or bags of fruit instead.

Retract shoulder blades

Slightly bend knees

1

Stand with your feet shoulder-width apart and hold a dumbbell in each hand. Engage your core and bend over to 45 degrees from the hips. Let your arms hang in front of you, palms facing your knees.

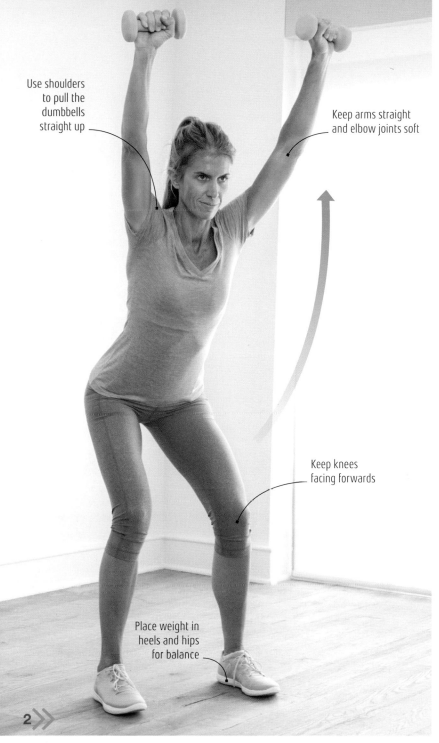

Use shoulders to pull the dumbbells straight up

Keep arms straight and elbow joints soft

Keep knees facing forwards

Place weight in heels and hips for balance

2 ≫

Engage the muscles in your shoulders and upper back to raise the dumbbells straight up until your arms are aligned with your spine. Keep your arms straight and only move from the shoulder joints.

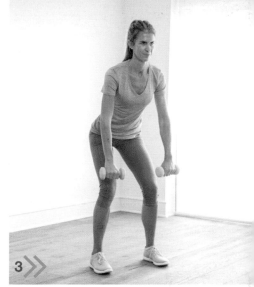

3 ≫

In a controlled manner, lower the dumbbells to the starting position, keeping your arms straight. Continue to repeat the exercise with quick, controlled movements for the time given in your workout.

/// MAKE IT **easier**

If it is difficult to raise the dumbbells overhead or if you feel pain in your shoulder joints, do the exercise without weights.

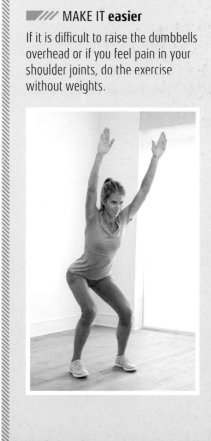

Upright external rotation

Weakness and lack of mobility in the rotator cuffs can cause pain throughout the day and make it difficult to sleep. Use this controlled movement to strengthen and improve mobility in all of the muscles that support your arms and shoulders.

IMPROVES
//// Posture
//// **Strength**
//// **Mobility**

WHAT YOU NEED
Dumbbells

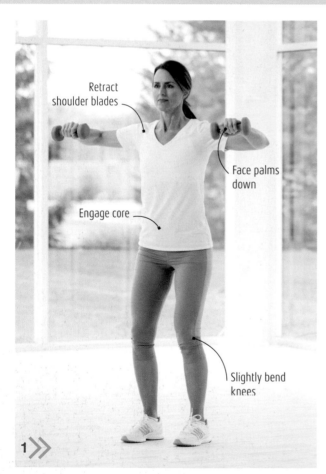

Retract shoulder blades

Face palms down

Engage core

Slightly bend knees

1 >>

Stand with your feet shoulder-width apart, slightly bend your knees, and hold a dumbbell in each hand. Raise your upper arms out to the side at shoulder height, bend your elbows to 90 degrees, and position your forearms parallel to the ground.

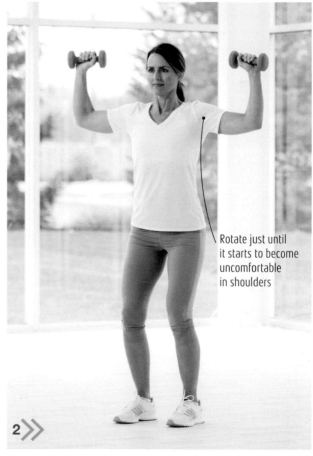

Rotate just until it starts to become uncomfortable in shoulders

2 >>

Engage your upper back and shoulder muscles to pull the dumbbells back. Rotate your arms up until you reach the top of your range of motion, keeping your upper arms parallel to the ground. Continue to retract your shoulder blades.

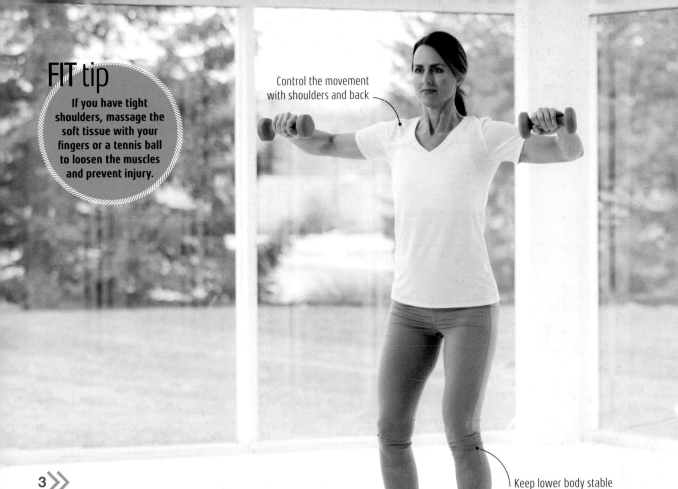

FIT tip

If you have tight shoulders, massage the soft tissue with your fingers or a tennis ball to loosen the muscles and prevent injury.

Control the movement with shoulders and back

Keep lower body stable and isolate movement to shoulders

3 ≫

In a controlled manner, rotate your arms forwards to lower the dumbbells back to the starting position. Maintain the 90-degree bend in your elbows and keep your upper back engaged. Continue to repeat the exercise for the time given in your workout.

//// **MAKE IT easier**

If it is difficult or painful to raise the dumbbells, do the exercise without weights.

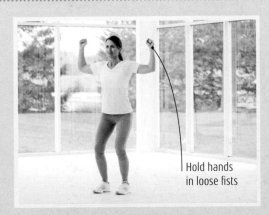

Hold hands in loose fists

IMPROVES
/// **Posture**
/// **Strength**
/// **Stability**

WHAT YOU NEED
Dumbbells

Bent row and hammer curl

Activities such as playing with children require you to bend over and pick up weight. Prepare for these movements with this quick and controlled compound exercise that improves total-body stability and strengthens your back and biceps.

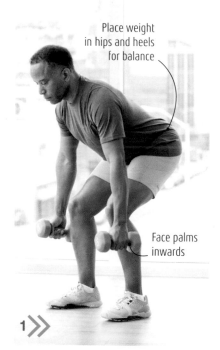

Place weight in hips and heels for balance

Face palms inwards

1 >>

Stand with your feet shoulder-width apart and hold a dumbbell in each hand. Bend over to 45 degrees from the hips and slightly bend your knees. Let your arms hang straight down.

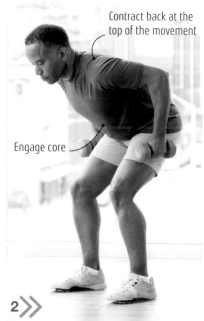

Contract back at the top of the movement

Engage core

2 >>

Retract your shoulder blades and pull the dumbbells up and back from your elbows until your upper arms are parallel to the ground. Keep your elbows tight to your body.

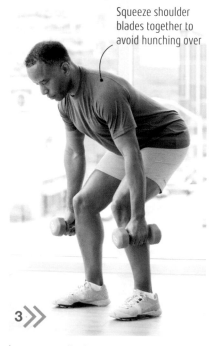

Squeeze shoulder blades together to avoid hunching over

3 >>

In a controlled manner, lower the dumbbells back to the starting position, keeping your back muscles engaged. Allow a slight bend in your elbow joints and keep your core firm.

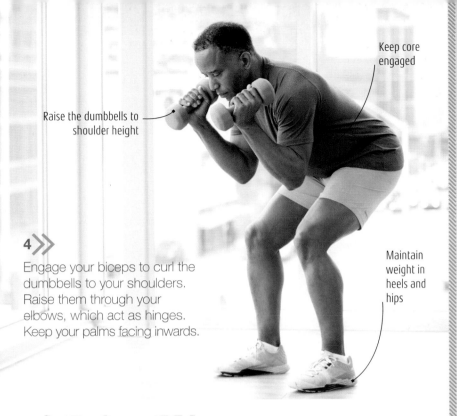

Keep core
engaged

Raise the dumbbells to
shoulder height

Maintain
weight in
heels and
hips

4 »

Engage your biceps to curl the
dumbbells to your shoulders.
Raise them through your
elbows, which act as hinges.
Keep your palms facing inwards.

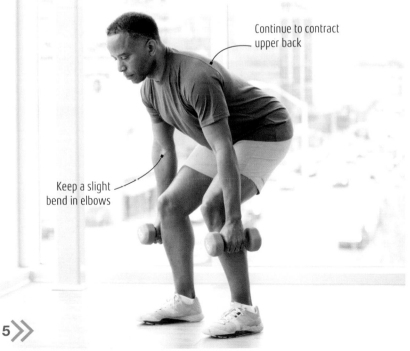

Continue to contract
upper back

Keep a slight
bend in elbows

5 »

In a controlled manner, extend your elbows and lower
the dumbbells to the starting position. Repeat the
sequence for the time given in your workout.

//// MAKE IT **easier**

To lessen the strain on your
lower back, sit on the edge
of a chair while performing
the exercise.

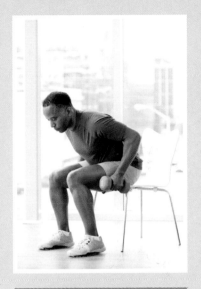

//// MAKE IT **harder**

To improve your balance, do
the exercise while balanced
on one leg. Bend your knees
and suspend your raised foot
behind you. Spend equal time
balancing on each leg.

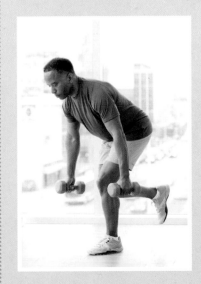

IMPROVES

/// Posture

/// Strength

/// Mobility

WHAT YOU NEED
Wall

Wall angel

Proper posture requires back strength and chest flexibility. Many daily activities such as sitting at a desk or driving a car can weaken and tighten these muscles, but you can use this stretching exercise to reverse the effects. By elongating your chest and building your back muscles, this exercise will open a tight chest and back and help fix rounded shoulders.

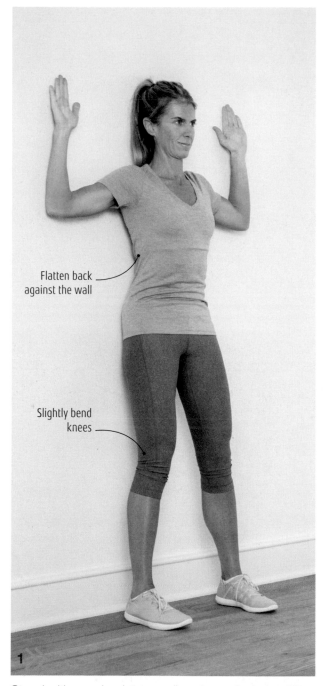

Flatten back against the wall

Slightly bend knees

1

Stand with your back to a wall and your feet shoulder-width apart, about 10cm (4in) from the wall. Rest your back and head against the wall. Raise your arms to the side, bend your elbows, and rest the backs of your arms and hands against the wall.

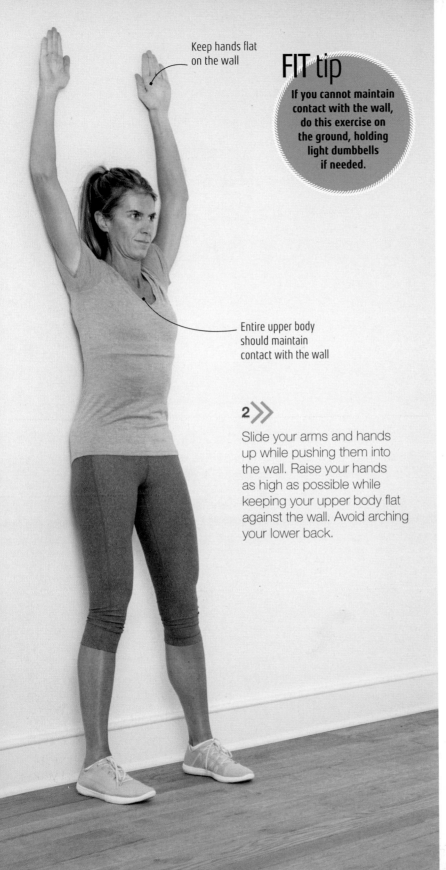

Keep hands flat on the wall

FIT tip

If you cannot maintain contact with the wall, do this exercise on the ground, holding light dumbbells if needed.

Entire upper body should maintain contact with the wall

2 ≫

Slide your arms and hands up while pushing them into the wall. Raise your hands as high as possible while keeping your upper body flat against the wall. Avoid arching your lower back.

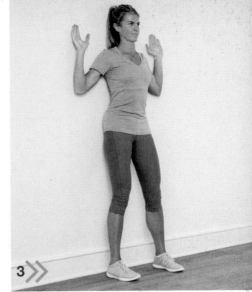

3 ≫

Using your back muscles, pull your arms back to the starting position. Continue to push your arms and hands into the wall, and repeat the exercise for the time given.

//// **MAKE IT harder**

To increase resistance to your back, add a resistance band. Hold one side of the band in each hand, place it behind your head, and pull the band apart. Maintain constant tension by pulling as you do the exercise.

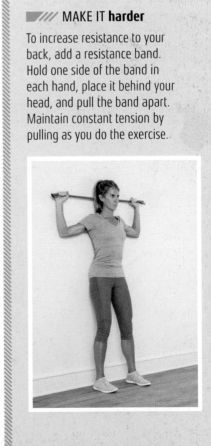

One-arm lift

IMPROVES
/// Posture
/// Strength
/// Stability
/// Mobility

WHAT YOU NEED
Dumbbell

Your back is one of the most powerful muscle groups in your body, so it is important to train it with exercises like this snatch so that your posture is better and your full-body movements are more efficient and stable. Perform this quick power move to develop a strong upper and lower back.

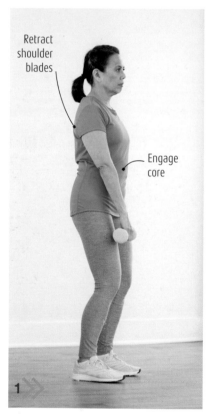

Retract shoulder blades

Engage core

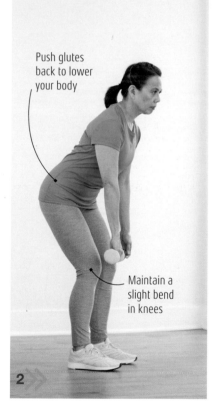

Push glutes back to lower your body

Maintain a slight bend in knees

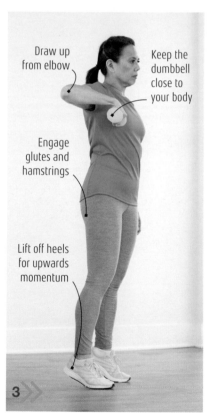

Draw up from elbow

Keep the dumbbell close to your body

Engage glutes and hamstrings

Lift off heels for upwards momentum

1 Stand with your feet shoulder-width apart. Hold a dumbbell in your right hand, palm facing you, and let your right arm hang in front of you. Let your left arm hang at your side, and slightly bend your knees.

2 Push your hips back and bend over at the waist until the dumbbell is at knee height. Keep your back straight and shoulders retracted. Let your left arm hang neutrally, and keep your core engaged.

3 In one quick motion, push your hips forwards to return to an upright position, pull your right arm up from the elbow until your elbow is at shoulder height, and rise briefly onto the balls of your feet.

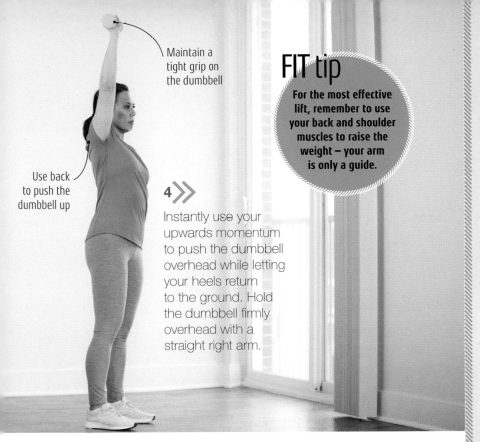

Maintain a tight grip on the dumbbell

Use back to push the dumbbell up

FIT tip

For the most effective lift, remember to use your back and shoulder muscles to raise the weight – your arm is only a guide.

4 ≫

Instantly use your upwards momentum to push the dumbbell overhead while letting your heels return to the ground. Hold the dumbbell firmly overhead with a straight right arm.

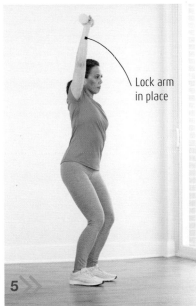

Lock arm in place

5 ≫

Immediately bend your knees and hips to absorb the weight of the dumbbell. Maintain a flat back and avoid hunching forwards.

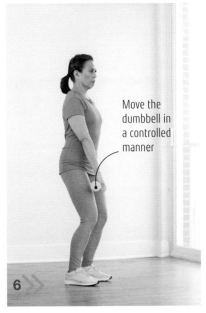

Move the dumbbell in a controlled manner

6 ≫

Return to the starting position. Repeat for the time given in your workout. Spend half the time on your right arm, then swap to your left arm.

▰/// MAKE IT easier

For a simpler movement, do steps 1–3, then lower the dumbbell to the starting position in a controlled manner without pushing the dumbbell overhead.

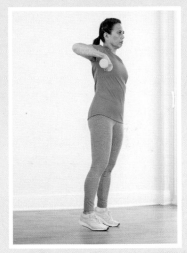

▰/// MAKE IT harder

To strengthen your legs, in step 5, sit back until your thighs are parallel to the ground. Stand back up before lowering the dumbbell.

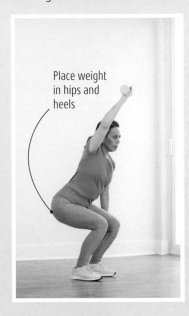

Place weight in hips and heels

Bird dog

Training your abdominals but neglecting your lower back will eventually lead to poor stability and alignment. Use this yoga exercise to strengthen your core and stabilize the lower back for upper- and lower-body movements.

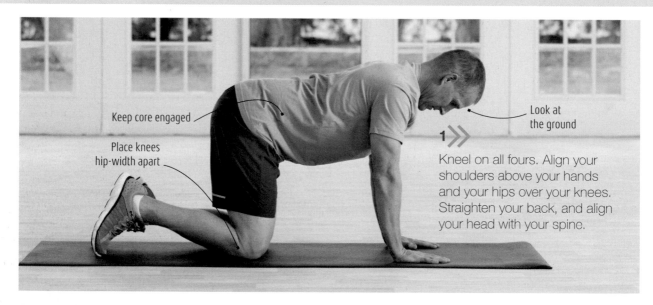

Keep core engaged

Place knees hip-width apart

Look at the ground

1 »

Kneel on all fours. Align your shoulders above your hands and your hips over your knees. Straighten your back, and align your head with your spine.

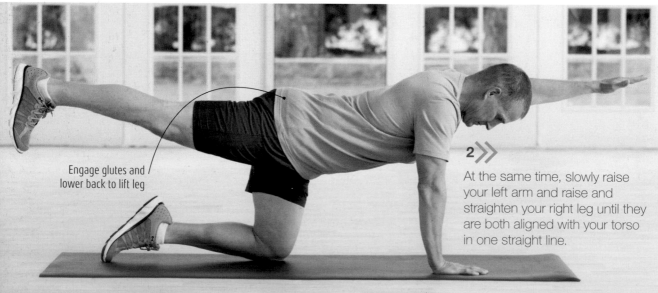

Engage glutes and lower back to lift leg

2 »

At the same time, slowly raise your left arm and raise and straighten your right leg until they are both aligned with your torso in one straight line.

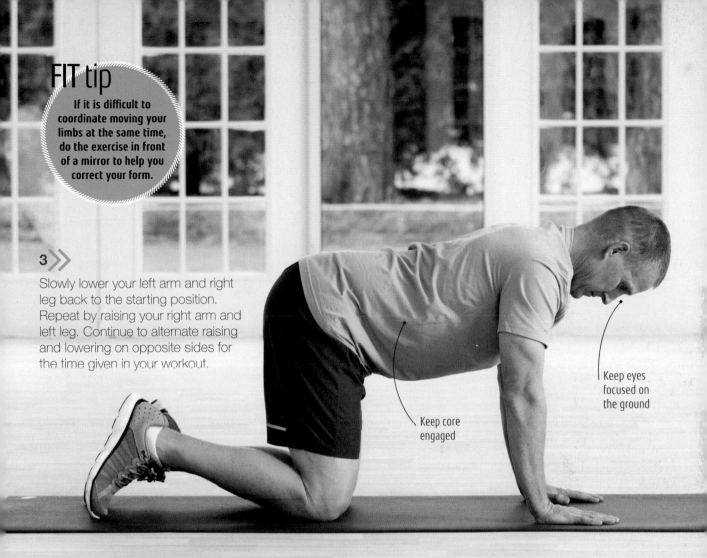

FIT tip

If it is difficult to coordinate moving your limbs at the same time, do the exercise in front of a mirror to help you correct your form.

3 »

Slowly lower your left arm and right leg back to the starting position. Repeat by raising your right arm and left leg. Continue to alternate raising and lowering on opposite sides for the time given in your workout.

Keep eyes focused on the ground

Keep core engaged

//// MAKE IT **easier**

To lessen the pressure on your lower back, in step 2, leave your hands on the ground and extend only your leg.

//// MAKE IT **harder**

To strengthen your abdominals, in step 3, do a crunch by pulling your elbow and knee to each other before returning to all fours.

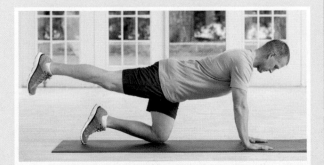

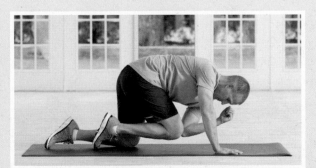

IMPROVES
- ▰/// Posture
- ▰/// Strength
- ▰/// Stability
- ▰/// Endurance

WHAT YOU NEED
Mat

High plank row

The plank is one of the best exercises for building your core strength, but it is also great for strengthening your back, glutes, and hamstrings. By combining the plank with a controlled rowing movement, this exercise develops your balance and helps improve posture.

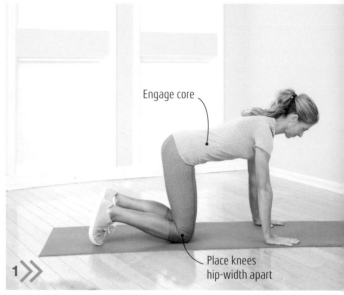

Engage core

Place knees hip-width apart

1 ⟫

Kneel on all fours. Align your shoulders above your hands with your fingers facing forwards. Straighten your back and align your head with your spine. Look at the ground and retract your shoulder blades.

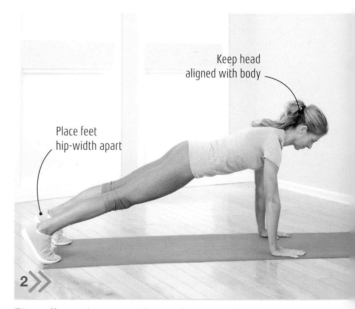

Keep head aligned with body

Place feet hip-width apart

2 ⟫

Rise off your knees and onto the balls of your feet. Walk your feet back into a plank position to form a straight line from head to heels. Evenly distribute your weight between the balls of your feet and your hands. Do not let your hips sink down or rise up.

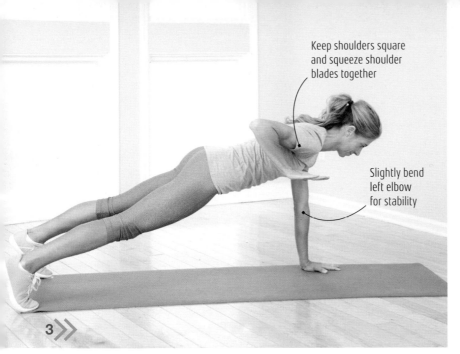

Keep shoulders square and squeeze shoulder blades together

Slightly bend left elbow for stability

3 ≫

In a controlled manner, pull your right arm back from your elbow, keeping your elbow close to your body and palm facing down. Contract your upper back at the top of the movement. Maintain a stable base with your left arm.

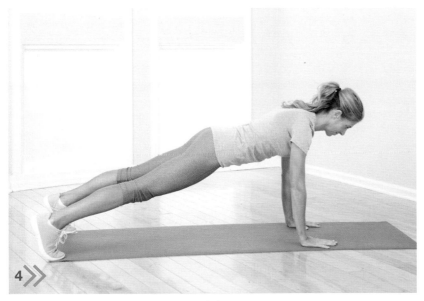

4 ≫

In a controlled manner, return your right arm to the starting position and redistribute your weight to both hands. Repeat the exercise with your left arm. Continue to alternate rowing with each arm for the time given in your workout.

MAKE IT **easier**

To reduce the strain on your core, remain on your knees instead of getting into a plank position. Lower your hips down until your upper body is at about a 45-degree angle to the ground.

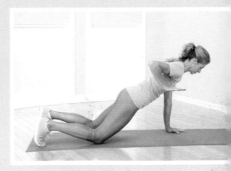

MAKE IT **harder**

To increase resistance to your back, hold a dumbbell in each hand and use the handles to support your upper body. Pull the dumbbells back from your elbow.

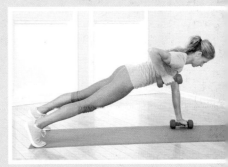

Stiff-leg deadlift and shrug

IMPROVES

/// Posture
/// Strength
/// Stability
/// Mobility

WHAT YOU NEED
Dumbbells

Strong muscles in the back of your body are the foundation for safe and efficient movement during daily activities. This swift, compound pulling exercise works your glutes, back muscles, and hamstrings to improve your overall stability.

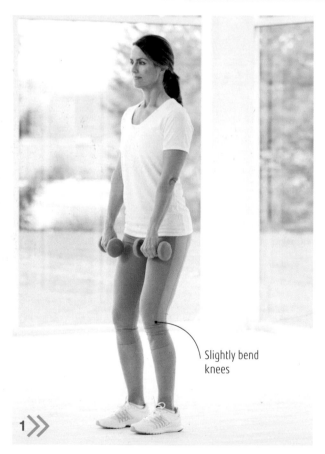

Slightly bend knees

1 »

Stand with your feet shoulder-width apart. Hold a dumbbell in each hand, palms facing you, and let your arms hang in front of you. Engage your core and retract your shoulder blades.

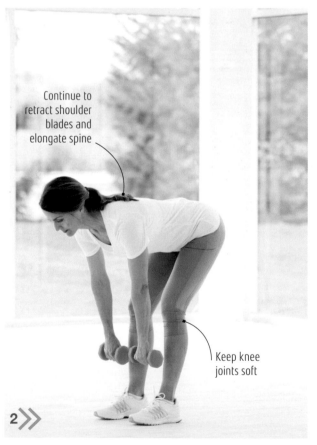

Continue to retract shoulder blades and elongate spine

Keep knee joints soft

2 »

In a quick and controlled manner, push your hips back and bend at the waist until your upper body is parallel to the ground. Let your arms move downwards, suspending the dumbbells above your feet.

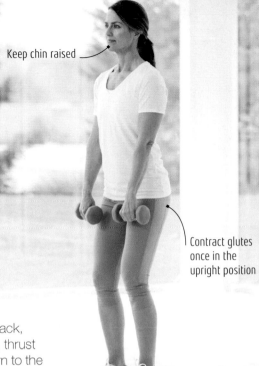

Keep chin raised

Contract glutes once in the upright position

3 »

Using your glutes, lower back, and hamstrings for power, thrust your hips forwards to return to the starting position. Let your arms travel back up with your body.

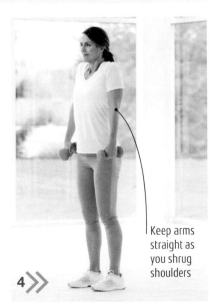

Keep arms straight as you shrug shoulders

4 »

In one motion, move the dumbbells to your sides by rotating your arms outwards, and use your upper-back muscles to raise your shoulders as high as possible towards your ears.

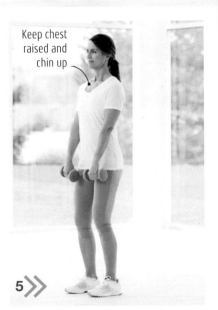

Keep chest raised and chin up

5 »

Controlling the movement with your back, push the dumbbells down and rotate your arms to the starting position. Repeat the sequence for the time given.

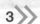 **MAKE IT easier**

If you have limited hamstring flexibility, in step 2, push your hips back and bend at your waist until the dumbbells are at your knees.

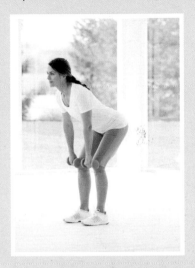

MAKE IT harder

To improve your balance, in step 2, lift your right foot off the ground and slowly kick your leg back as you bend over. Repeat the exercise by raising your left leg.

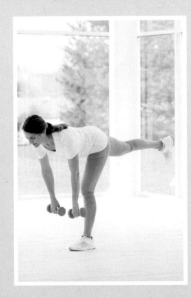

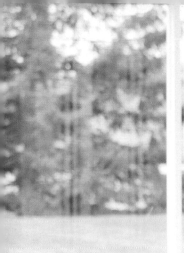

IMPROVES
/// Posture
/// Strength
/// Stability
/// Endurance

WHAT YOU NEED
Dumbbells

Seesaw row

From running to cycling, most endurance exercises are lower-body dominant, but it is important not to neglect your upper body. Perform this quick and dynamic upper-body pull to add variety to your workout and improve your upper-body endurance. Because one arm is suspended in front of you while the other is pulling up, this unique exercise also recruits your core for balance.

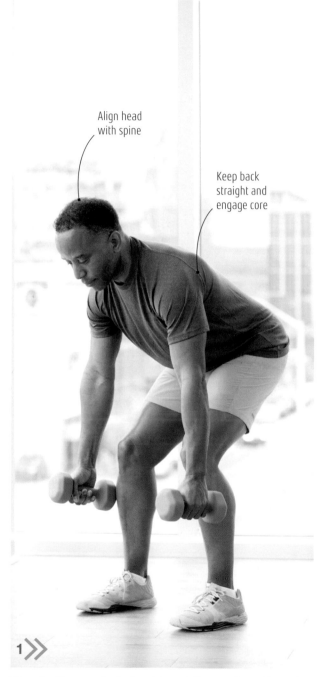

Align head with spine

Keep back straight and engage core

1 》

Stand with your feet shoulder-width apart and bend over to 45 degrees from the waist. Hold a dumbbell in each hand, palms facing each other, and let your arms hang straight down. Distribute your weight between your heels and hips.

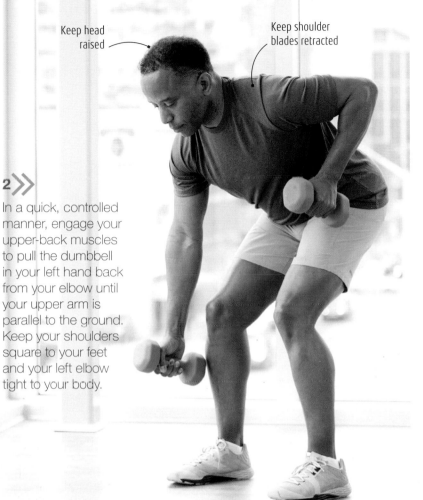

Keep head raised

Keep shoulder blades retracted

Continue to engage core

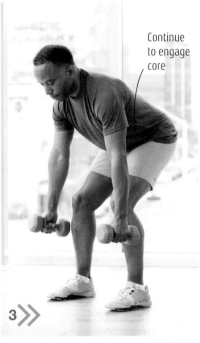

2 ≫

In a quick, controlled manner, engage your upper-back muscles to pull the dumbbell in your left hand back from your elbow until your upper arm is parallel to the ground. Keep your shoulders square to your feet and your left elbow tight to your body.

3 ≫

In a controlled manner, lower the dumbbell to the starting position, then immediately pull the dumbbell in your right hand back from your elbow. Continue to alternate rowing with each arm for the time given in your workout.

▟/// MAKE IT **easier**

If it is difficult to maintain balance, sit on the edge of a chair while performing the exercise.

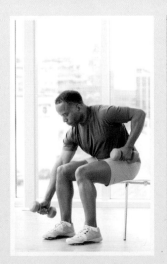

▟/// MAKE IT **harder**

To work your abdominals, in step 2, while you are pulling, use your core to twist your body towards the dumbbell.

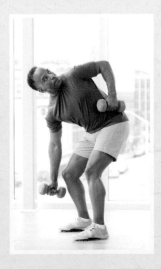

IMPROVES
/// **Strength**
/// **Stability**

WHAT YOU NEED
Dumbbell

Curl from one leg

Nearly every movement you make employs your balance system, recruiting the processes needed to send sensory information from your brain to your muscles. Use this quick and controlled curl to promote healthy body awareness as well as strengthen your biceps.

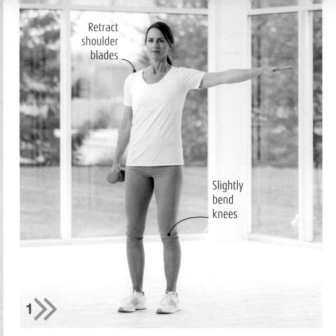

Retract shoulder blades

Slightly bend knees

1 >>

Stand with your feet shoulder-width apart. Hold a dumbbell in your right hand and let your right arm hang at your side. Extend your left arm out to your side, palm facing the ground. Engage your core.

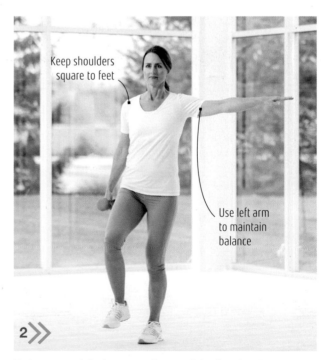

Keep shoulders square to feet

Use left arm to maintain balance

2 >>

Raise your right knee until your right foot is about 13cm (5in) from the ground, and transfer your weight to your left heel and your hips.

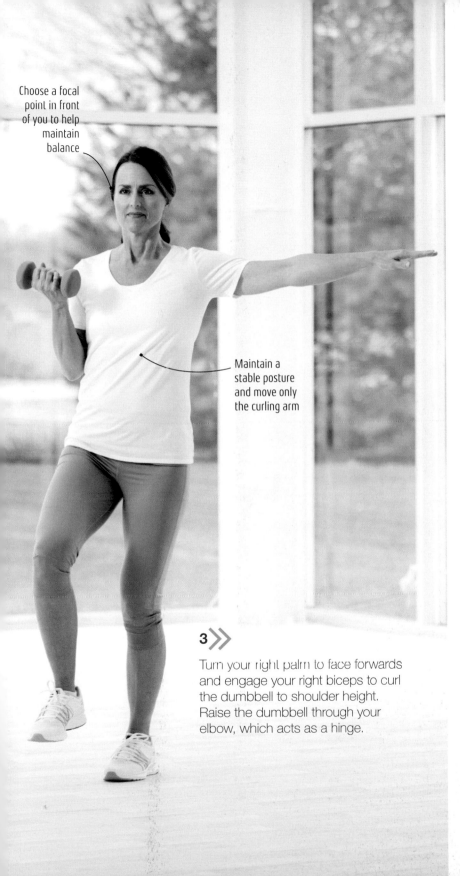

Choose a focal point in front of you to help maintain balance

Maintain a stable posture and move only the curling arm

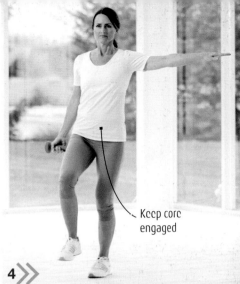

Keep core engaged

4 »

In a quick, controlled manner, lower the dumbbell straight down. Without lowering your right foot, repeat the curl. Spend half the given time curling with your right arm, then reverse your stance and curl with your left arm.

3 »

Turn your right palm to face forwards and engage your right biceps to curl the dumbbell to shoulder height. Raise the dumbbell through your elbow, which acts as a hinge.

//// **MAKE IT easier**

For additional support, rest your extended hand on a chair or wall. Use the support when needed, but try not to rely on it too much.

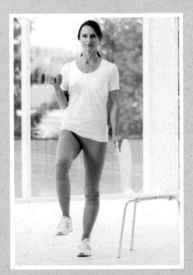

Standing elbow to knee

IMPROVES

■>/// **Strength**

■/// **Stability**

/// Mobility

■/// **Endurance**

WHAT YOU NEED
No equipment needed

A firm core protects and stabilizes your spine, but it requires more than just crunches to strengthen these muscles. Do this exercise swiftly to increase your rotational ability and build your abdominals so your spine is secure and your torso remains effortlessly upright.

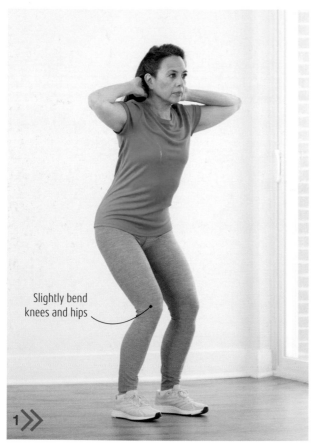

Slightly bend knees and hips

1 >>

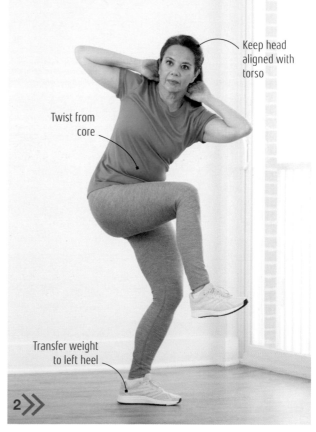

Keep head aligned with torso

Twist from core

Transfer weight to left heel

2 >>

Stand with your feet shoulder-width apart. Place your hands on the back of your head and point your elbows out to your sides. Engage your core, retract your shoulder blades, and raise your chin.

Transfer your weight to your left heel, raise your right knee and pull it towards the centre of your body, and bring your left elbow towards your right knee by rotating your core. Maintain a bend in your left knee.

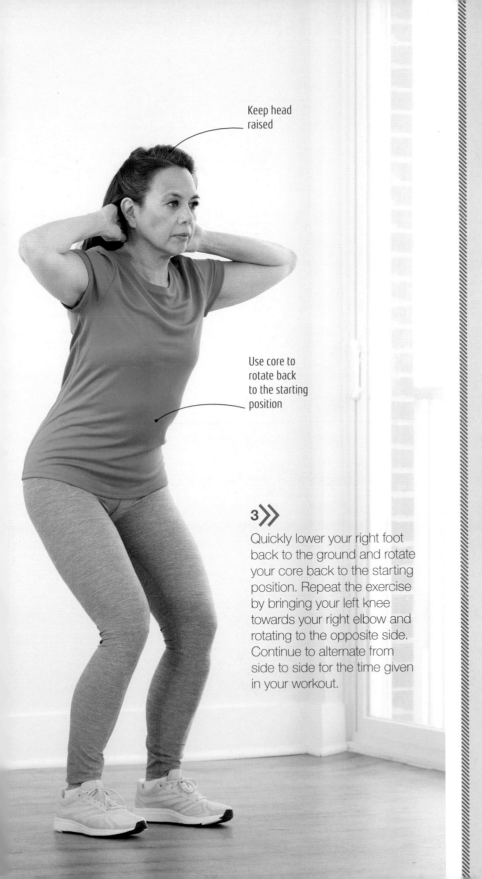

Keep head raised

Use core to rotate back to the starting position

3 »

Quickly lower your right foot back to the ground and rotate your core back to the starting position. Repeat the exercise by bringing your left knee towards your right elbow and rotating to the opposite side. Continue to alternate from side to side for the time given in your workout.

▰/// MAKE IT **easier**

If it is difficult to maintain balance, extend your arms out to your sides rather than placing them behind your head. Rotate your arms and core on a horizontal plane.

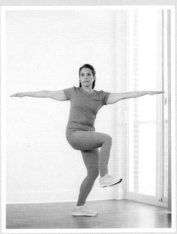

▰/// MAKE IT **harder**

To develop power in your legs, in step 2, jump up off the balls of your feet as you bring your knee towards your elbow. In step 3, land softly on the balls of your feet.

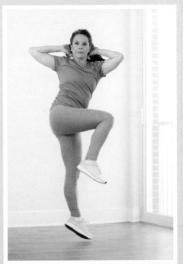

Split stance runners

IMPROVES

▰/// Strength

▰/// Stability

/// Mobility

▰/// Endurance

WHAT YOU NEED

No equipment needed

Whether you are running half marathons or taking walks around your neighbourhood, strong upper-body movement will immensely improve your body's efficiency. Vigorously perform this drill to practise proper walking mechanics and strengthen your upper-body muscles.

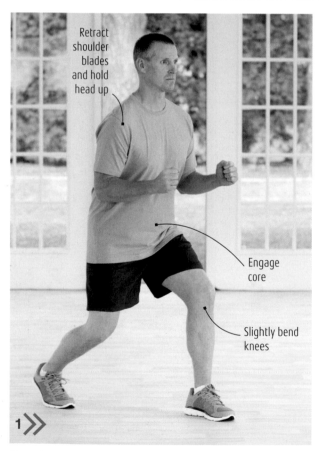

Retract shoulder blades and hold head up

Engage core

Slightly bend knees

1 >>

Stand with your feet shoulder-width apart. Step your right leg back into a staggered stance and rise up onto the ball of your right foot. Bend both elbows to 90 degrees, position your forearms in front of you, and hold your hands in loose fists.

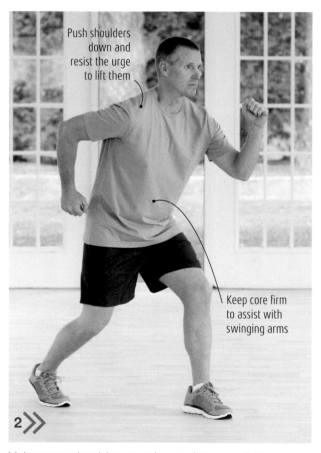

Push shoulders down and resist the urge to lift them

Keep core firm to assist with swinging arms

2 >>

Using your shoulder muscles, swing your right arm back until your right hand is just behind your body, and swing your left arm forwards until your left hand is at chin height. Maintain a 90-degree bend in both elbows and keep your elbows close to your body.

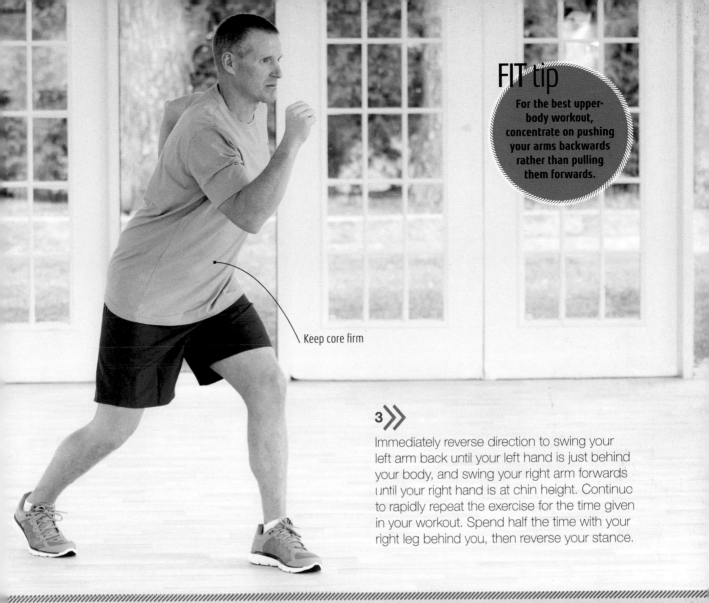

FIT tip

For the best upper-body workout, concentrate on pushing your arms backwards rather than pulling them forwards.

Keep core firm

3 »

Immediately reverse direction to swing your left arm back until your left hand is just behind your body, and swing your right arm forwards until your right hand is at chin height. Continue to rapidly repeat the exercise for the time given in your workout. Spend half the time with your right leg behind you, then reverse your stance.

/// MAKE IT **easier**

If it is difficult to maintain balance, stand with your feet shoulder-width apart rather than in the staggered stance.

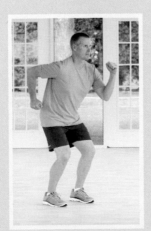

/// MAKE IT **harder**

To increase resistance to your shoulders, hold a dumbbell in each hand as you swing your arms.

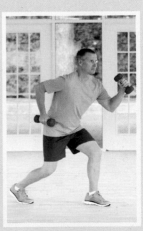

Wood chop

Rotational movements require you to activate smaller stabilizing muscles such as the hip flexors, which are not typically worked by other exercises. This fast-paced squat awakens those muscles to improve your balance.

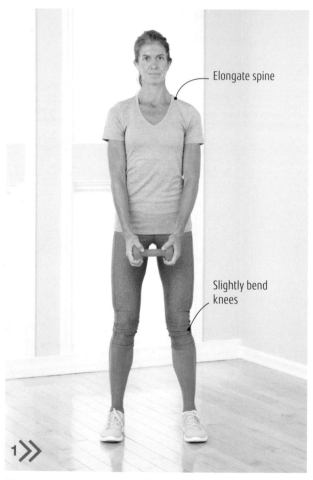

Elongate spine

Slightly bend knees

1 ⟫

Stand with your feet shoulder-width apart. Hold the ends of a dumbbell with both hands, and let your arms hang straight down in front of you. Engage your core and retract your shoulder blades.

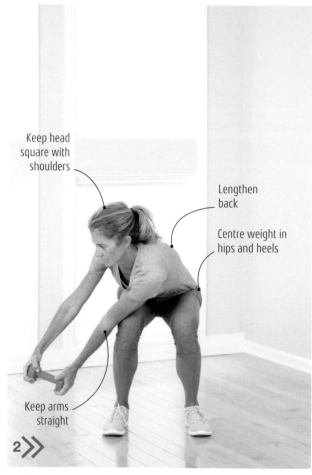

Keep head square with shoulders

Lengthen back

Centre weight in hips and heels

Keep arms straight

2 ⟫

Push your glutes back and bend at your hips and knees to sit back into a squat until your thighs are parallel to the ground. Simultaneously rotate your core to bring the dumbbell to the outside of your right leg.

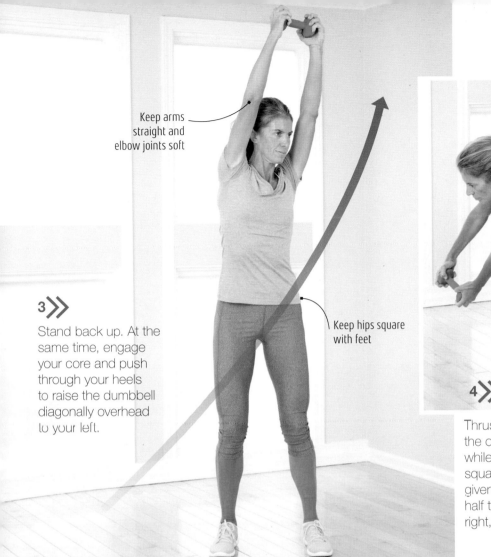

Keep arms straight and elbow joints soft

Keep hips square with feet

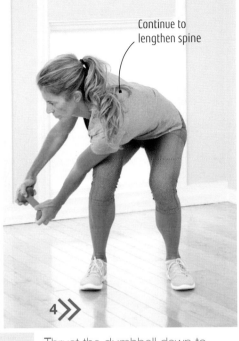

Continue to lengthen spine

3 »

Stand back up. At the same time, engage your core and push through your heels to raise the dumbbell diagonally overhead to your left.

4 »

Thrust the dumbbell down to the outside of your right leg while entering into the next squat. Repeat for the time given in your workout. Spend half the time thrusting to your right, then repeat to your left.

/// MAKE IT **easier**

To decrease resistance to your core, do the exercise without a dumbbell. Keep your hands and arms straight, and hold them shoulder-width apart.

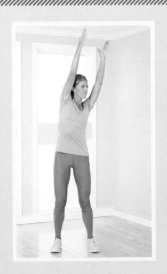

/// MAKE IT **harder**

To increase resistance to your thighs, in step 1, step your right leg back into a staggered stance. In step 2, drop your back knee into a lunge rather than squatting. Remain in the staggered stance for each repetition. Reverse your stance halfway through.

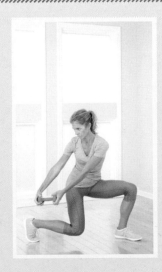

IMPROVES
///// **Posture**
///// **Strength**
///// **Stability**
///// **Mobility**
///// **Endurance**

WHAT YOU NEED
Dumbbell

Knee chop

Training your abdominals while standing up engages more muscles and burns more calories than most ground-based exercises. Perform this standing core exercise swiftly to work your entire body, boost your endurance, burn fat, and significantly improve your posture.

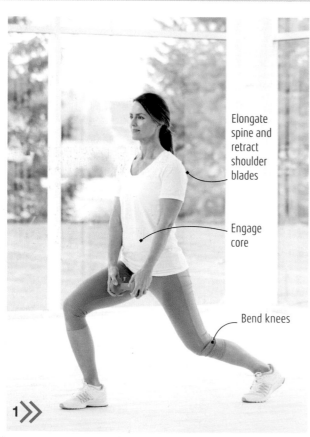

Elongate spine and retract shoulder blades

Engage core

Bend knees

1 ➤➤ Stand with your feet shoulder-width apart, step your left leg back into a staggered stance, and rise up onto the ball of your left foot. Hold the ends of a dumbbell with both hands, and let your arms hang straight down in front of you.

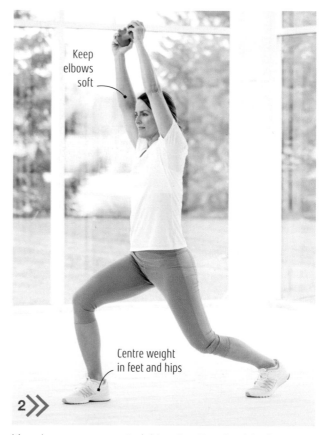

Keep elbows soft

Centre weight in feet and hips

2 ➤➤ Keeping your arms straight, raise the dumbbell diagonally overhead to your right. Do not lock your elbow joints. Look straight ahead and maintain an upright posture. Keep your core engaged.

Continue to retract
shoulder blades

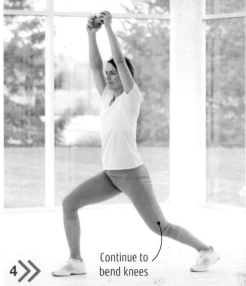

4 »

Continue to
bend knees

Return to the staggered stance,
and raise the dumbbell diagonally
overhead to the right. Repeat the
exercise for the time given in your
workout. Spend half the time
raising your right leg, then swap
to your left leg.

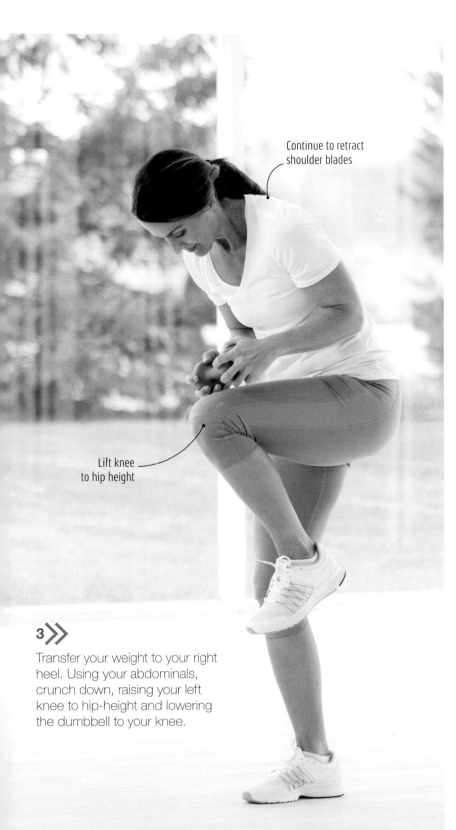

Lift knee
to hip height

3 »

Transfer your weight to your right
heel. Using your abdominals,
crunch down, raising your left
knee to hip-height and lowering
the dumbbell to your knee.

▰/// **MAKE IT easier**

If it is difficult to maintain
balance, do the exercise
without a dumbbell, and
hold your hands in fists.

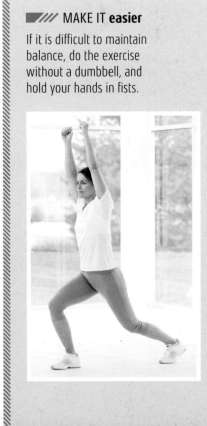

IMPROVES
- ▰/// **Strength**
- ▰/// **Stability**
- ▱/// Mobility
- ▰/// **Endurance**

WHAT YOU NEED
Dumbbells

Side-to-side punch

You do not have to be a boxer to benefit from cardio boxing. This punching sequence can improve heart health, develop core strength, burn calories, and build shoulder muscles. You might also find this exercise to be a remarkable stress reliever.

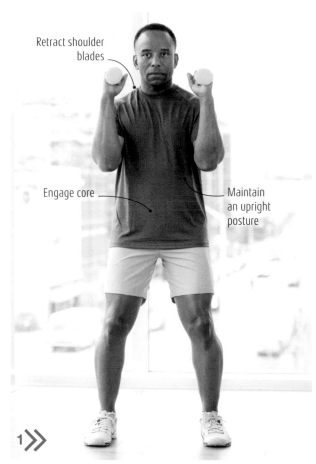

Retract shoulder blades

Engage core

Maintain an upright posture

1 ≫

Stand with your feet shoulder-width apart. Hold a dumbbell in each hand, raise them to chin-height with your palms facing each other, and tuck your elbows to your sides. Slightly bend your knees and hips.

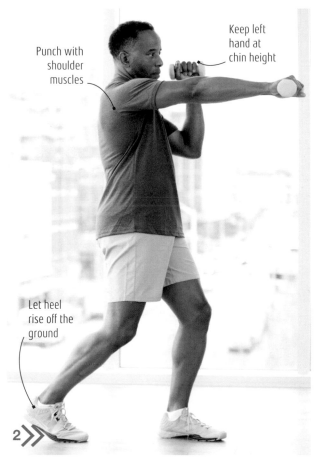

Keep left hand at chin height

Punch with shoulder muscles

Let heel rise off the ground

2 ≫

Engage your core and hips to rotate your body 90 degrees to the left, letting your feet rotate with you. Simultaneously punch your right arm out and rotate your arm so your palm faces the ground.

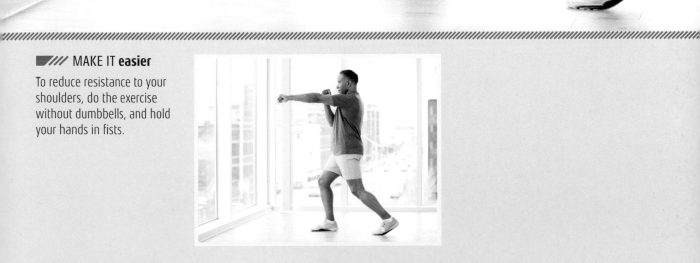

FIT tip

To protect your elbow joints from injury, always retract your punch just before reaching a full extension.

Keep core engaged

3

Powerfully rotate 180 degrees to the right, while at the same pulling your right arm back to the starting position and punching with your left arm. Continue to swiftly rotate your body 180 degrees and alternate punching with each arm for the time given in your workout.

///// MAKE IT **easier**

To reduce resistance to your shoulders, do the exercise without dumbbells, and hold your hands in fists.

IMPROVES
■//// **Strength**
■//// **Stability**
//// **Mobility**
■//// **Endurance**

WHAT YOU NEED
Dumbbell

Standing twist

Spinal flexibility is just as important as muscle flexibility. A mobile spine promotes healthy posture, better enabling you to comfortably lift heavy objects or perform throwing motions. Use this swift, rotational, core-strengthening exercise to restore natural mobility to your spine, relieve chronic back pain, and reduce your chances of injury.

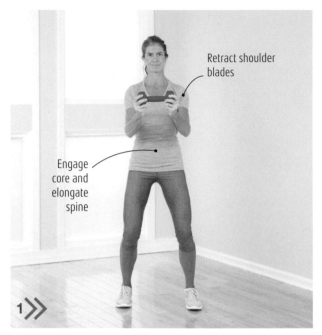

Retract shoulder blades

Engage core and elongate spine

1 »

Stand with your feet shoulder-width apart. Hold the ends of a dumbbell with both hands, bend your elbows to 90 degrees, and raise the dumbbell to chest height. Slightly bend your knees and hips.

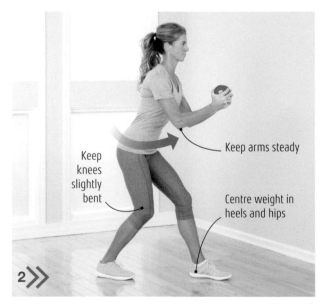

Keep knees slightly bent

Keep arms steady

Centre weight in heels and hips

2 »

Using your hips and core for momentum, quickly pivot your feet and rotate your upper body 90 degrees to the left. Keep the dumbbell aligned with your chest and let your arms travel with you.

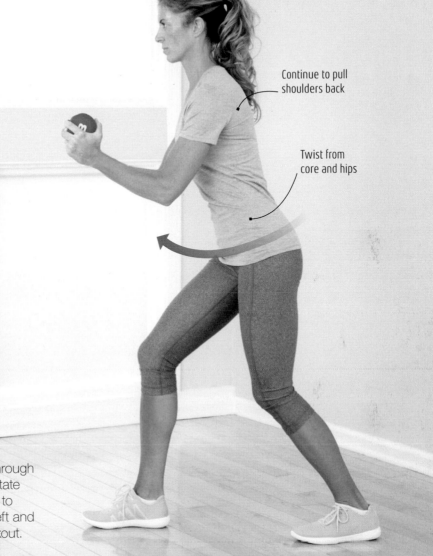

FIT tip

If the aches in your back stubbornly persist, the Bird dog and Hip-ups are great additions to the Standing twist.

Continue to pull shoulders back

Twist from core and hips

3 »

Keeping your arms steady, push through your heels and pivot your feet to rotate 180 degrees to the right. Continue to rapidly twist 180 degrees to your left and right for the time given in your workout.

///// MAKE IT **easier**

If it is difficult to maintain balance, hold your arms in the same position, but do the exercise without a dumbbell.

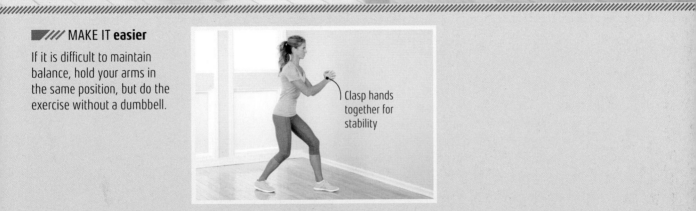

Clasp hands together for stability

Standing oblique rotation

Torso strength and mobility will stabilize your spine and make all your movements more efficient. Do this rotational exercise to strengthen your abdominals and lower back, take pressure off your spine, and help you more safely do activities such as cleaning or gardening.

IMPROVES
/// Posture
/// **Strength**
/// **Stability**
/// Mobility

WHAT YOU NEED
Dumbbell

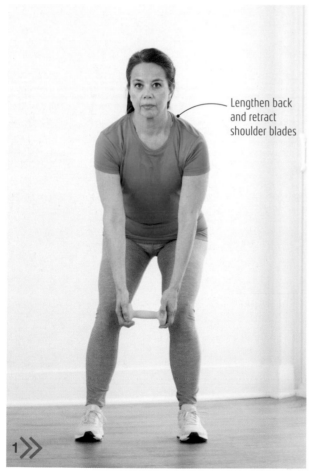

Lengthen back and retract shoulder blades

1 >> Stand with your feet shoulder-width apart and bend over to 45 degrees from the hips. Hold the ends of a dumbbell with both hands and let your arms hang straight down in front of you. Slightly bend your knees.

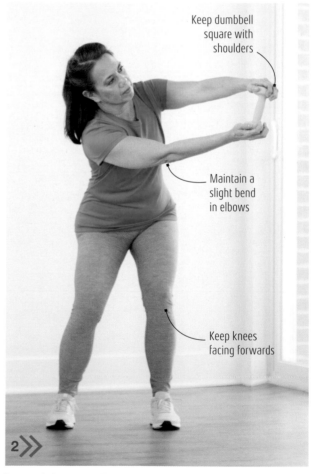

Keep dumbbell square with shoulders

Maintain a slight bend in elbows

Keep knees facing forwards

2 >> In a quick, controlled manner, use your hips and core to rotate your torso and arms 90 degrees to the left. Move your head along with your shoulders and follow the dumbbell with your eyes.

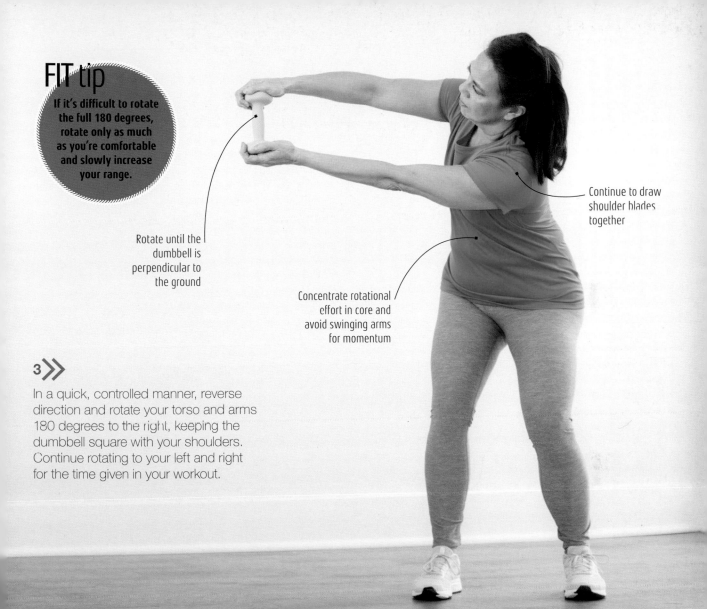

FIT tip

If it's difficult to rotate the full 180 degrees, rotate only as much as you're comfortable and slowly increase your range.

Rotate until the dumbbell is perpendicular to the ground

Continue to draw shoulder blades together

Concentrate rotational effort in core and avoid swinging arms for momentum

3 »

In a quick, controlled manner, reverse direction and rotate your torso and arms 180 degrees to the right, keeping the dumbbell square with your shoulders. Continue rotating to your left and right for the time given in your workout.

▰▰▰ MAKE IT easier

To reduce pressure on your spine, do the exercise without a dumbbell, and hold your hands in fists.

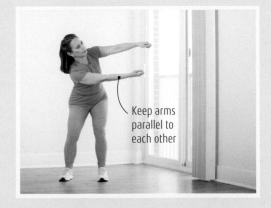

Keep arms parallel to each other

Rotational goblet squat

Squatting is actually very functional – we squat naturally as babies, but many lose the ability after years of frequently sitting in unnatural positions. Perform this quick and controlled exercise to strengthen your legs and core and restore your natural ability to squat.

IMPROVES
/// Strength
/// Stability
/// Mobility
/// Endurance

WHAT YOU NEED
Dumbbell

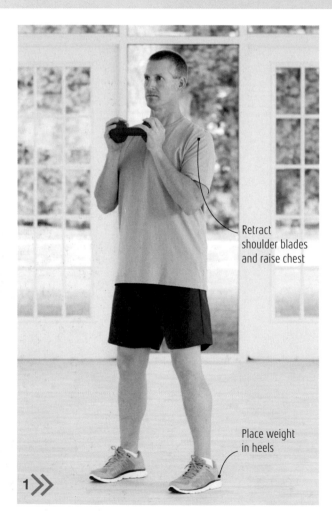

Retract shoulder blades and raise chest

Place weight in heels

1 》》 Stand with your feet shoulder-width apart and hold the ends of a dumbbell with both hands. Raise the dumbbell to your chest. Engage your core.

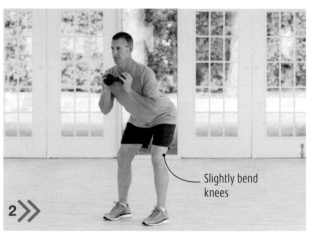

Slightly bend knees

2 》》 Push your glutes back and bend at your hips. Keep your back long and straight, and keep your knees facing forwards. Hold your head up.

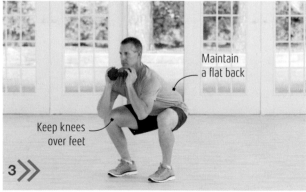

Maintain a flat back

Keep knees over feet

3 》》 Without moving the dumbbell, bend your knees and sit back into a squat until your thighs are parallel to the ground. Keep your weight in your heels and hips.

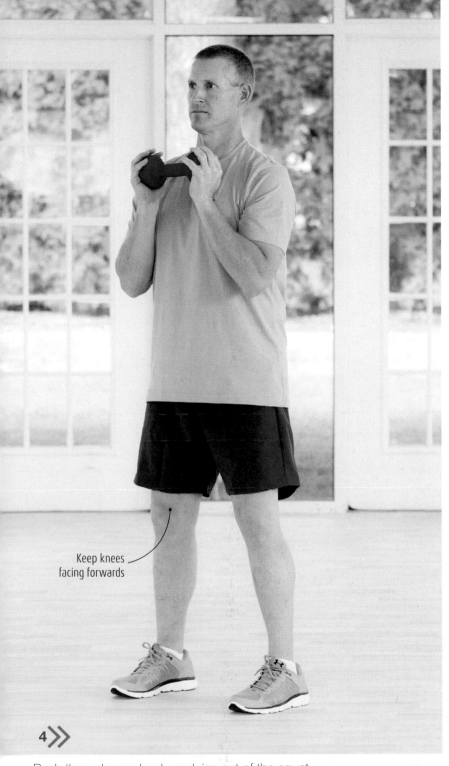

Keep knees
facing forwards

4 ▶▶

Push through your heels and rise out of the squat
until your legs are straight. Keep your head aligned
with your spine and your chest raised.

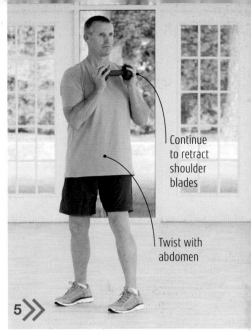

Continue
to retract
shoulder
blades

Twist with
abdomen

5 ▶▶

Using your core, rotate your torso
90 degrees to the left, letting your
arms move with you. Then return
to the starting position. Alternate
rotating to your right and left for
the time given in your workout.

▰/// MAKE IT **easier**

If it is difficult to maintain
balance, place a chair behind
you and squat until you lightly
touch the chair. Do the exercise
without a dumbbell, holding
your hands in loose fists.

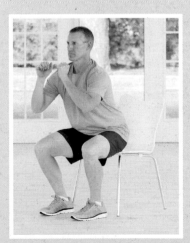

Crossover toe touch

IMPROVES

/// Posture
/// Strength
/// Stability
/// Mobility
/// Endurance

WHAT YOU NEED
No equipment needed

In order for your upper and lower body to work together harmoniously, you must train your abdominals and your lower back together. Energetically perform this exercise to work these muscles simultaneously and develop better stability and body awareness.

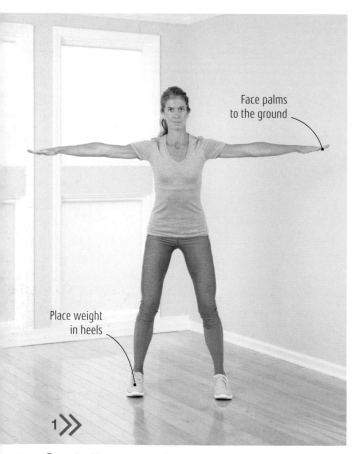

Face palms to the ground

Place weight in heels

1 »

Stand with your feet slightly wider than shoulder-width apart and extend your arms straight out to your sides, palms facing down. Retract your shoulder blades and engage your core. Slightly bend your knees and hips.

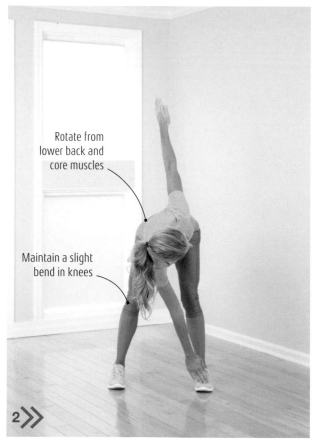

Rotate from lower back and core muscles

Maintain a slight bend in knees

2 »

Keeping your arms straight and rotating from your core, reach your right hand down to touch your left foot by bending at your hips and pushing your glutes back. Keep your head up.

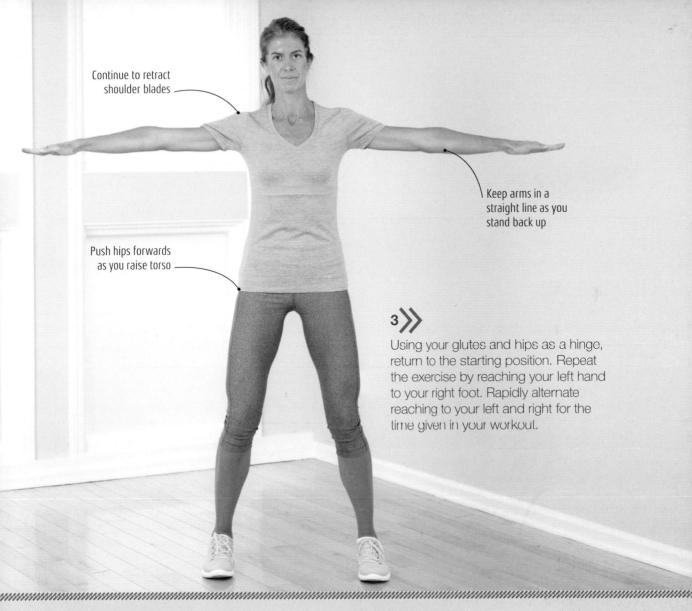

Continue to retract shoulder blades

Keep arms in a straight line as you stand back up

Push hips forwards as you raise torso

3 »

Using your glutes and hips as a hinge, return to the starting position. Repeat the exercise by reaching your left hand to your right foot. Rapidly alternate reaching to your left and right for the time given in your workout.

▰/// MAKE IT **easier**

If flexibility in your hamstrings is limited, reach to your knees rather than your feet.

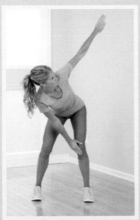

▰/// MAKE IT **harder**

To increase resistance to your shoulders and core, hold a light dumbbell in each hand.

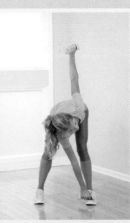

IMPROVES

/// Posture
/// **Strength**
/// **Stability**
/// Mobility

WHAT YOU NEED
Mat

High plank reach-through and fly

Planks condition your body to use your abdominals for stabilization. Plus, they are safer than crunches because they don't require you to flex your spine. Perform this rotational variation to improve your core stability and strength.

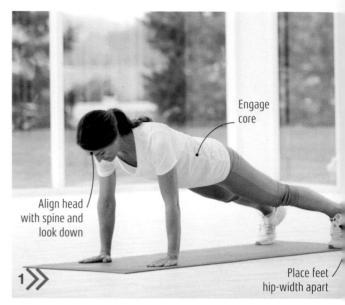

Engage core

Align head with spine and look down

Place feet hip-width apart

1 »

Kneel on all fours and align your shoulders above your hands, fingers facing forwards. Rise off your knees and onto the balls of your feet, and walk your feet back into a modified plank position to form a straight line from your head to heels.

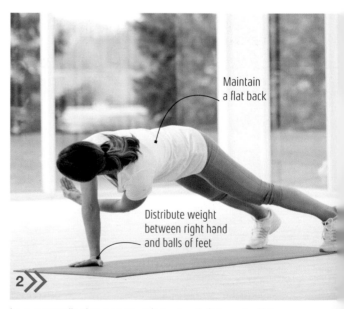

Maintain a flat back

Distribute weight between right hand and balls of feet

2 »

In a controlled manner, raise your left hand off the ground. Rotating from your core, reach your left arm under your right arm and across your body as if you are wrapping your arm around a tree trunk.

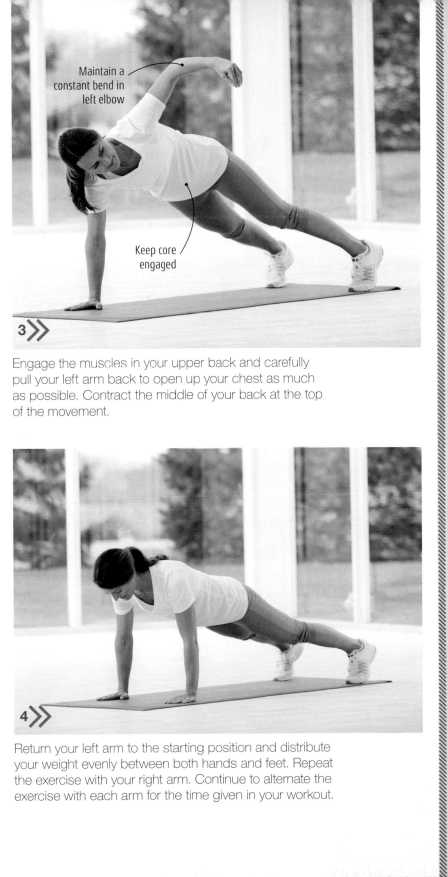

Maintain a constant bend in left elbow

Keep core engaged

3 »

Engage the muscles in your upper back and carefully pull your left arm back to open up your chest as much as possible. Contract the middle of your back at the top of the movement.

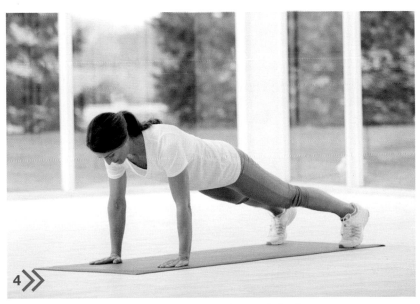

4 »

Return your left arm to the starting position and distribute your weight evenly between both hands and feet. Repeat the exercise with your right arm. Continue to alternate the exercise with each arm for the time given in your workout.

▰▰/// MAKE IT easier

If it is difficult to maintain balance, remain on your knees instead of getting into a plank position. Lower your hips until your upper body is about 45 degrees to the ground.

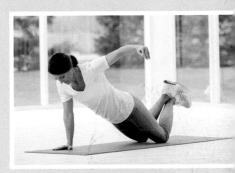

▰▰/// MAKE IT harder

To increase resistance, hold a dumbbell in your left hand and pull it back from your elbow. Spend half the time working your left side, then repeat on your right side.

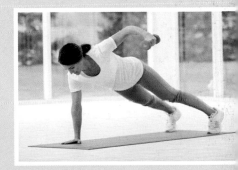

IMPROVES

/// Posture

/// **Strength**

/// **Stability**

/// Mobility

/// **Endurance**

WHAT YOU NEED

No equipment needed

Windmill

A variety of problems can cause lower-back pain, but many back injuries are avoidable by frequently doing preventative exercises. This controlled twisting exercise can improve the strength and flexibility of your abdominals and lower-back muscles so you can stay pain- and injury-free.

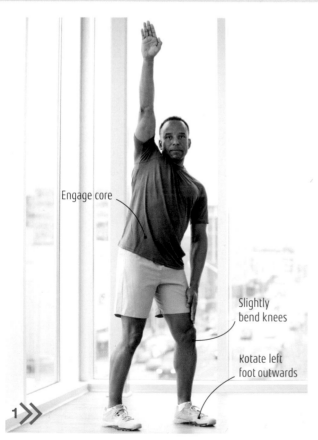

Engage core

Slightly bend knees

Rotate left foot outwards

1 >> Stand with your feet slightly wider than shoulder-width apart and angle your left foot out at about 45 degrees. Fully extend your right arm straight overhead and lock your elbow. Let your left arm hang straight down.

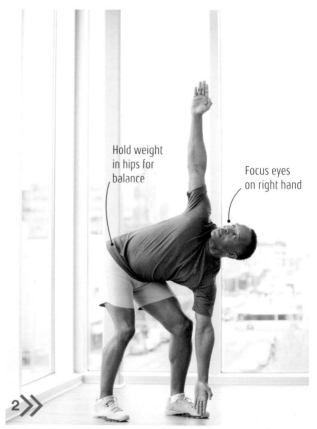

Hold weight in hips for balance

Focus eyes on right hand

2 >> Push your right hip out to your left and look up at your right hand. Keeping your back and arms straight and flexing your knees as necessary, bend to the left until your left hand touches the inside of your left foot.

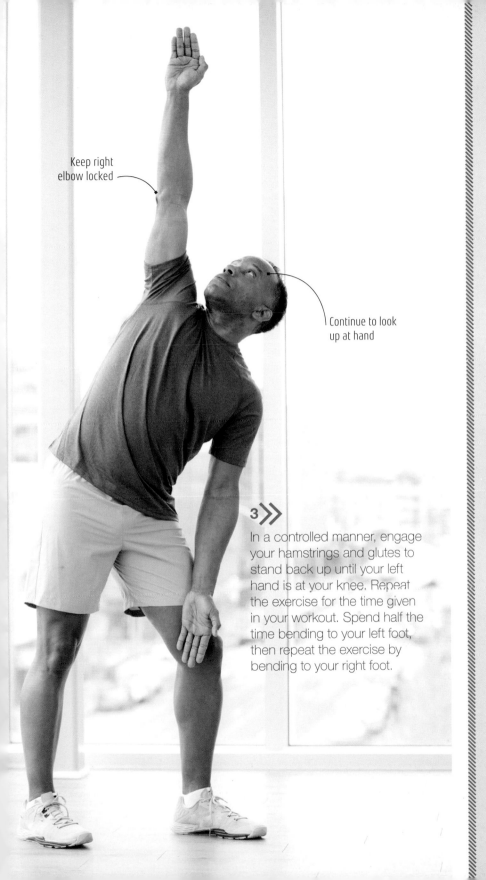

Keep right elbow locked

Continue to look up at hand

3 》

In a controlled manner, engage your hamstrings and glutes to stand back up until your left hand is at your knee. Repeat the exercise for the time given in your workout. Spend half the time bending to your left foot, then repeat the exercise by bending to your right foot.

▰▰/// MAKE IT **easier**

If your flexibility is limited, bend just until your hand reaches your knee.

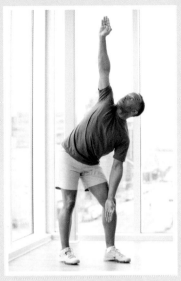

▰▰/// MAKE IT **harder**

To increase resistance to your shoulders and core, hold a dumbbell in your raised hand.

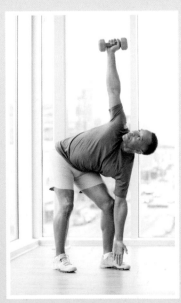

Over-the-shoulder squat

IMPROVES

▰/// Posture
▰/// **Strength**
▰/// Stability
/// Mobility
▰/// Endurance

WHAT YOU NEED
Dumbbell

Lower-back injuries are one of the most common reasons for visits to the doctor and often occur from improperly lifting objects. Practise safe lifting and develop your lower-body strength with this weighted squat, which helps stabilize your spine and improve total-body coordination.

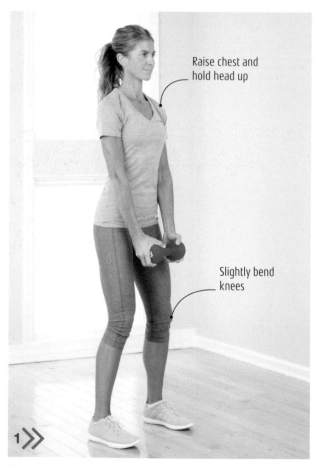

Raise chest and hold head up

Slightly bend knees

1 ⟫

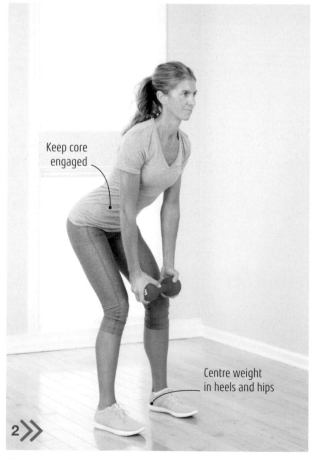

Keep core engaged

Centre weight in heels and hips

2 ⟫

Stand with your feet shoulder-width apart and hold the ends of a dumbbell with both hands. Let your arms hang straight down in front of you. Engage your core and retract your shoulder blades.

Push your glutes back and bend at your hips, letting the dumbbell move downwards. Keep your back straight and your knees pointed in the same direction as your feet. Hold your head up.

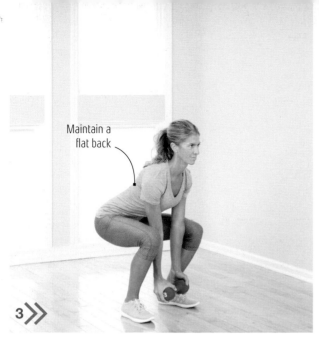

Maintain a
flat back

3 》》

In a quick, controlled manner, continue to bend your knees and sit back into a squat until your thighs are parallel to the ground. Let your arms hang straight down. Distribute your weight in your heels and hips.

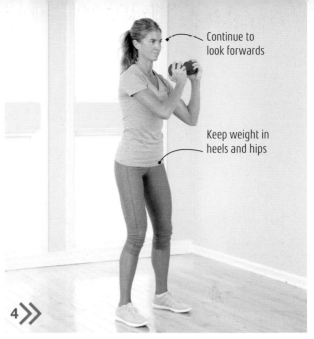

Continue to
look forwards

Keep weight in
heels and hips

4 》》

In one motion, quickly push through your heels to rise out of the squat until your legs are straight, and bend your elbows to swing the dumbbell up to your left shoulder.

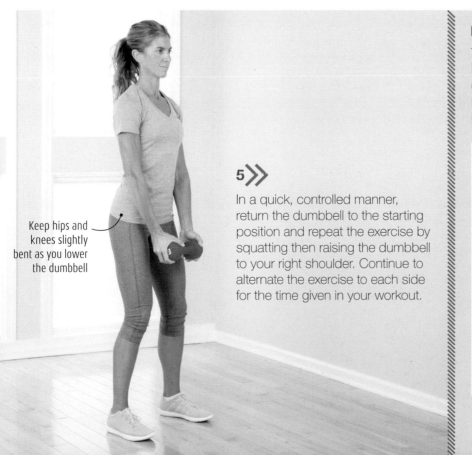

Keep hips and
knees slightly
bent as you lower
the dumbbell

5 》》

In a quick, controlled manner, return the dumbbell to the starting position and repeat the exercise by squatting then raising the dumbbell to your right shoulder. Continue to alternate the exercise to each side for the time given in your workout.

▰▰/// MAKE IT easier

To decrease resistance to your legs and shoulders, do the exercise without a dumbbell. Let your arms hang neutrally in front of you.

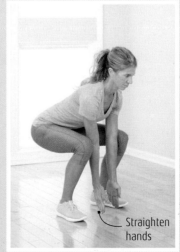

Straighten
hands

Diagonal chop

Most athletic movements involve a form of rotation, which requires your torso to generate and transfer power, but if your core is weak, it can lead to poor performance or injury. Enhance your core strength, stability, and power with this energy-intensive chopping exercise.

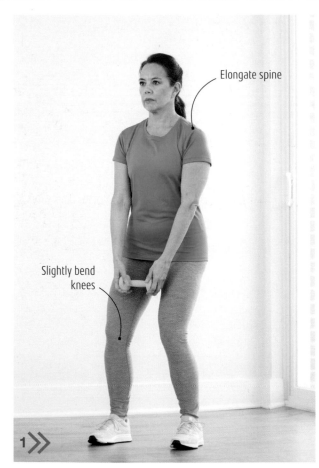

Elongate spine

Slightly bend knees

1 》》 Stand with your feet shoulder-width apart. Hold the ends of a dumbbell with both hands and let your arms hang straight down in front of you. Engage your core and retract your shoulder blades.

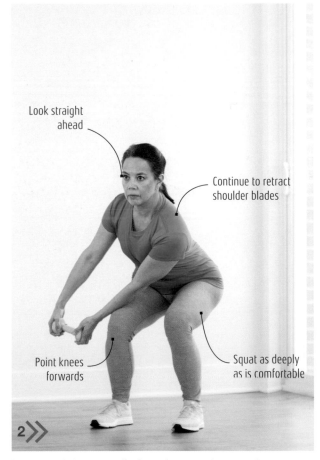

Look straight ahead

Continue to retract shoulder blades

Point knees forwards

Squat as deeply as is comfortable

2 》》 In one quick, controlled motion, push your glutes back and bend at your hips to sit back into a squat while rotating your core to lower the dumbbell to the outside of your right leg.

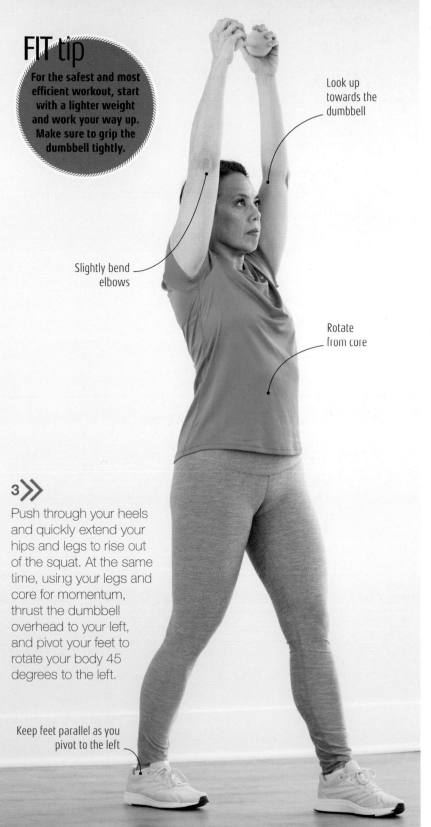

Look up towards the dumbbell

Slightly bend elbows

Rotate from core

3 »

Push through your heels and quickly extend your hips and legs to rise out of the squat. At the same time, using your legs and core for momentum, thrust the dumbbell overhead to your left, and pivot your feet to rotate your body 45 degrees to the left.

Keep feet parallel as you pivot to the left

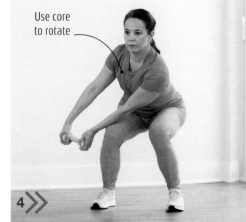

Use core to rotate

4 »

In a quick, controlled manner, enter into the next squat, pivot your feet to the starting position, and return the dumbbell to the outside of your right leg. Repeat for the time given. Spend half the time rotating to your left, then repeat to your right.

▰/// MAKE IT **easier**

To decrease the resistance to your legs, shoulders, and core, do the exercise without a dumbbell. Hold your hands in loose fists.

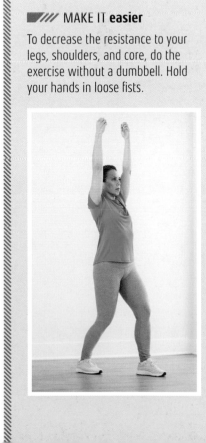

Suitcase squat

A lack of upper-leg strength can cause you to use your back muscles instead of your leg muscles for lifting heavy objects, which can lead to back injury. Perform this squat at a quick, controlled tempo to strengthen your quads and hamstrings, preparing you to safely lift anything from a suitcase to a child.

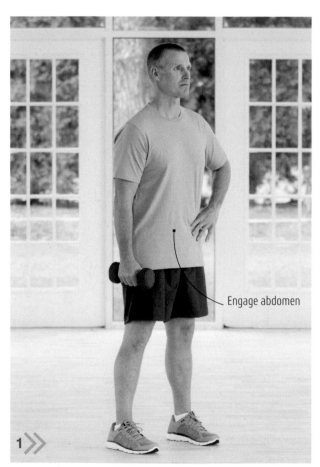

Engage abdomen

1 »

Stand with your feet shoulder-width apart. Hold a dumbbell in your right hand and let your right arm hang at your side. Place your left hand on your hip. Raise your head and retract your shoulder blades.

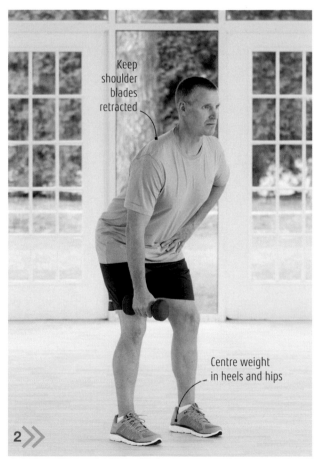

Keep shoulder blades retracted

Centre weight in heels and hips

2 »

Push your glutes back and bend at your hips, letting the dumbbell move downwards. Keep your back straight and keep your knees facing forwards. Hold your head up.

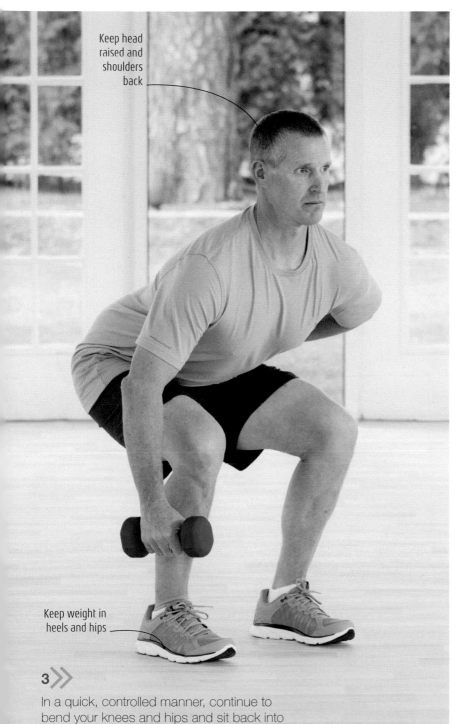

Keep head raised and shoulders back

Keep weight in heels and hips

3 ❯❯

In a quick, controlled manner, continue to bend your knees and hips and sit back into a squat until your thighs are parallel to the ground. Let your right arm hang straight down.

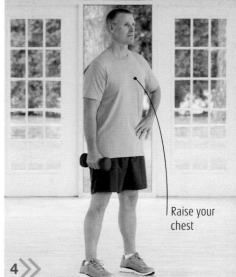

Raise your chest

4 ❯❯

Push through your heels and rise out of the squat. Repeat for the time given in your workout. Spend half the time with the dumbbell in your right hand, then switch to your left hand.

▰▰▱ **MAKE IT easier**

If it is difficult to balance, place a chair behind you and squat until your glutes lightly touch the chair.

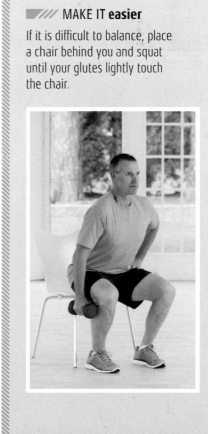

Walking reaching lunge

IMPROVES
▰/// **Strength**
▰/// **Stability**
/// Mobility
▰/// **Endurance**

WHAT YOU NEED
Dumbbells

Your nervous system controls your movements, so it is important to train it for complex actions like bending down and reaching. Perform this exercise to build a strong mind-body connection in addition to improving your total-body strength and stability.

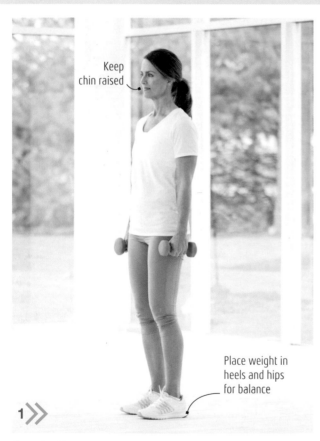

Keep chin raised

Place weight in heels and hips for balance

1 ≫

Stand with your feet shoulder-width apart. Hold a dumbbell in each hand, palms facing inwards, and let your arms hang at your sides. Engage your core and retract your shoulder blades.

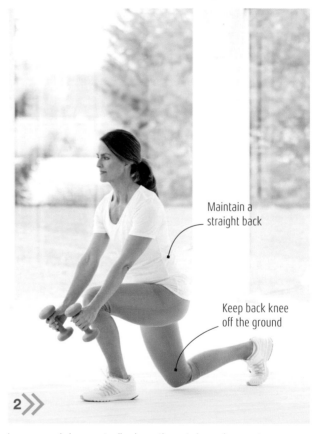

Maintain a straight back

Keep back knee off the ground

2 ≫

In one quick, controlled motion, take a long step forwards with your left leg, drop your right knee down until both knees are bent to 90 degrees, and extend the dumbbells down, past your left knee.

FIT tip

To improve stability for your hamstrings and glutes, stand in front of a short step and step your foot forwards onto the step.

Continue to retract shoulder blades

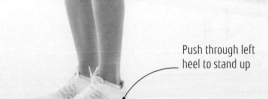

3 »

Quickly engage both legs to return to the starting position, while pulling the dumbbells back to your sides. Repeat the lunge by stepping forwards with your right leg. Continue to alternate lunging on each side for the time given in your workout.

Push through left heel to stand up

///// MAKE IT **easier**

To decrease the load on your legs, in step 1, step your right leg back into a staggered stance. In step 2, drop your right knee straight down into a lunge. Remain in the staggered stance for each repetition. Reverse your stance halfway through.

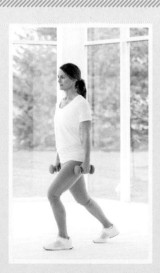

///// MAKE IT **harder**

To strengthen your arms, in step 3, after rising out of the lunge, engage your biceps to curl the dumbbells to shoulder height, then lower them again before doing the next lunge.

Face palms up

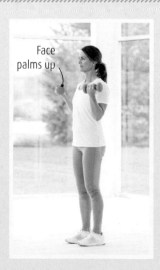

IMPROVES

/// **Posture**

/// **Strength**

/// **Stability**

/// **Mobility**

/// **Endurance**

WHAT YOU NEED
Dumbbell

Reverse lunge with twist

Everyday activities like walking, hiking, and climbing stairs require a unique combination of strength and stability. Perform this dynamic exercise to strengthen your legs and prepare your body to functionally tackle activities that demand lower-body stability.

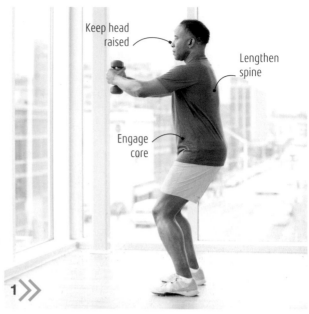

Keep head raised

Lengthen spine

Engage core

1 》

Stand with your feet shoulder-width apart. Hold a dumbbell with both hands. Raise the dumbbell to chest height and slightly bend your elbows out to your sides. Retract your shoulder blades.

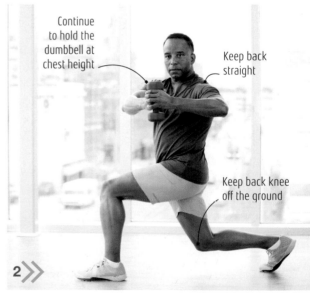

Continue to hold the dumbbell at chest height

Keep back straight

Keep back knee off the ground

2 》

In a controlled manner, step your right leg back and drop your right knee down until both knees are bent to 90 degrees. Simultaneously engage your core to rotate your upper body 90 degrees to the left.

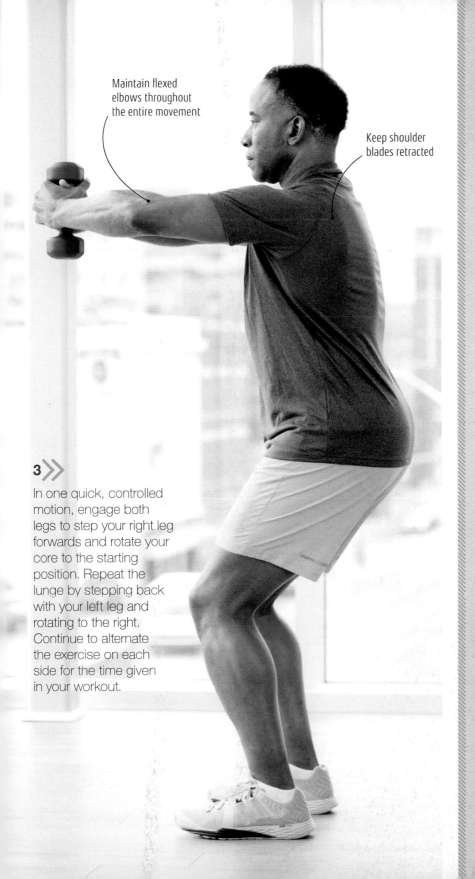

Maintain flexed elbows throughout the entire movement

Keep shoulder blades retracted

3 »

In one quick, controlled motion, engage both legs to step your right leg forwards and rotate your core to the starting position. Repeat the lunge by stepping back with your left leg and rotating to the right. Continue to alternate the exercise on each side for the time given in your workout.

///// **MAKE IT easier**

To decrease resistance to your legs, in step 1, step your left leg back into a staggered stance. In step 2, drop your left knee straight down into a lunge. Remain in the staggered stance for each repetition. Reverse your stance halfway through.

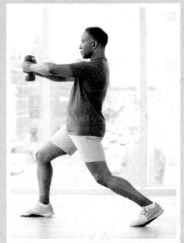

IMPROVES
- Posture
- Strength
- Stability
- Mobility
- Endurance

WHAT YOU NEED
Dumbbell

Posterior swing

This exercise strengthens your glutes, lower back, and hamstrings, doing wonders to counteract the negative effects of prolonged sitting. Use this powerful swinging movement to improve your posture and become more upright, open, and extended.

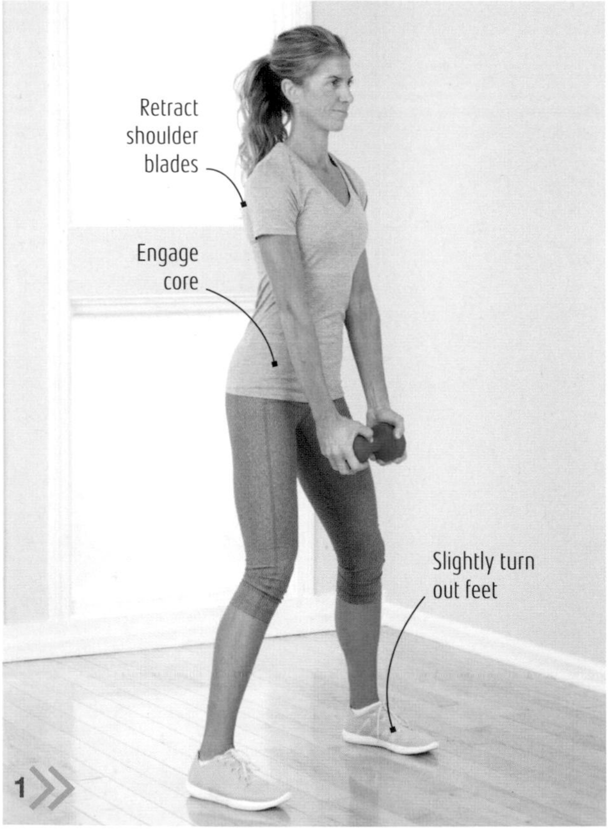
Retract
shoulder
blades
Engage
core
Slightly turn
out feet
1

Stand with your feet slightly wider than shoulder-width apart. Firmly hold the ends of a dumbbell with both hands and let your arms hang straight down in front of you. Slightly bend your knees and hips.

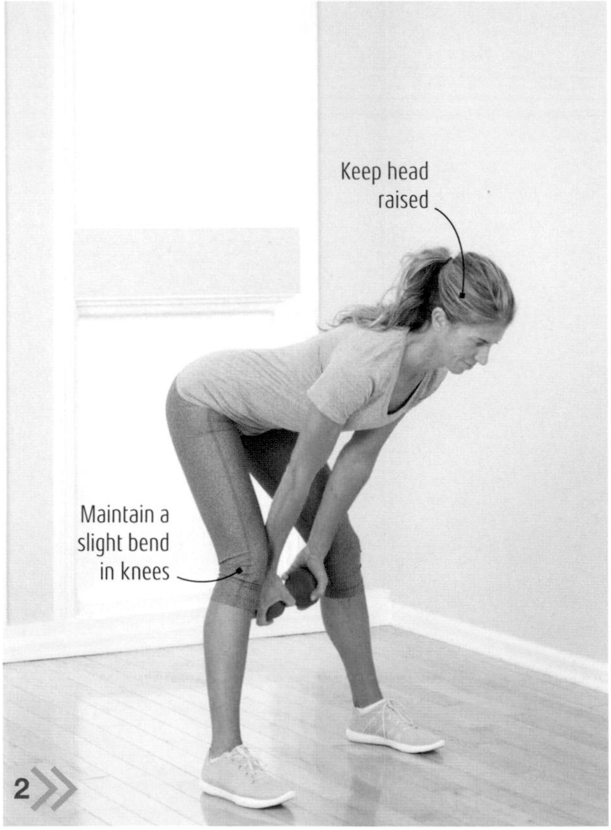
Keep head
raised
Maintain a
slight bend
in knees
2

Keeping your arms straight, quickly push your hips back, bend at the waist, and swing the dumbbell between your legs. Keep your back straight and avoid hunching forwards.

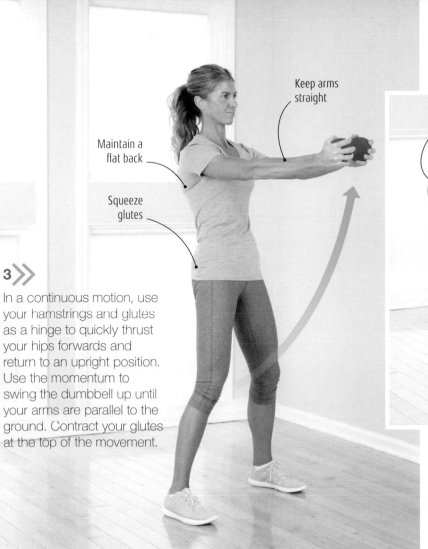

Keep arms
straight

Maintain a
flat back

Squeeze
glutes

3 »

In a continuous motion, use
your hamstrings and glutes
as a hinge to quickly thrust
your hips forwards and
return to an upright position.
Use the momentum to
swing the dumbbell up until
your arms are parallel to the
ground. Contract your glutes
at the top of the movement.

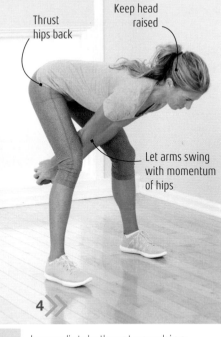

Thrust
hips back

Keep head
raised

Let arms swing
with momentum
of hips

4 »

Immediately thrust your hips
back and swing the dumbbell
between your legs for the next
repetition. Continue to repeat
the exercise swiftly for the time
given in your workout.

///// **MAKE IT easier**

To reduce resistance to
your back, do the exercise
without a dumbbell.
Instead, lock your fingers
together to make a fist.

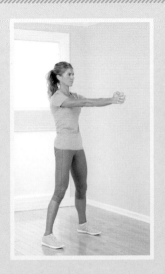

///// **MAKE IT harder**

To increase resistance to
your shoulders and upper
back, in step 3, swing the
dumbbell straight overhead.

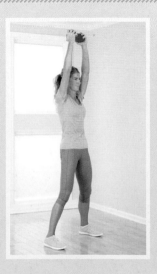

IMPROVES
/// **Posture**
/// **Strength**
/// **Stability**
/// **Mobility**

WHAT YOU NEED
Dumbbells

Good morning

Your glutes are the largest and most powerful muscle group in the body. Strong glutes can improve posture; alleviate lower back, hip, and knee pain; and even reduce bone density loss. Use this controlled power movement to strengthen these essential lower-body muscles.

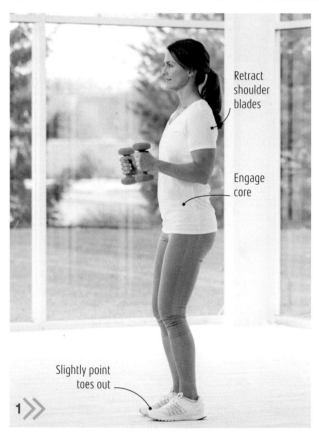

Retract shoulder blades

Engage core

Slightly point toes out

1 》》

Stand with your feet shoulder-width apart. Hold a dumbbell in each hand, palms facing inwards. Bend your elbows to 90 degrees, and raise the dumbbells to waist height. Slightly bend your knees and hips.

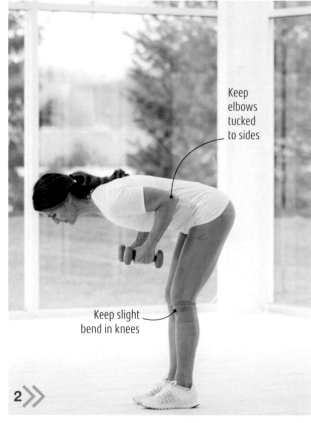

Keep elbows tucked to sides

Keep slight bend in knees

2 》》

Keeping your back straight, push your hips back and bend over at the waist until your upper body is parallel to the ground. Maintain a slight bend in your knees, but avoid lowering yourself with your knees.

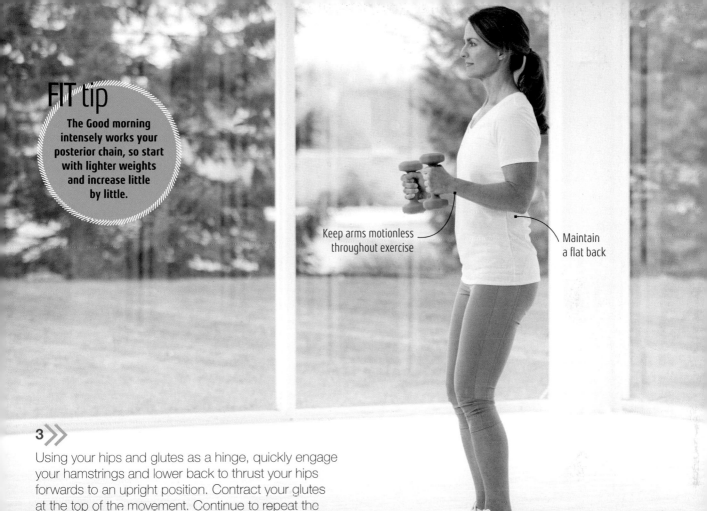

FIT tip

The Good morning intensely works your posterior chain, so start with lighter weights and increase little by little.

Keep arms motionless throughout exercise

Maintain a flat back

3 》》

Using your hips and glutes as a hinge, quickly engage your hamstrings and lower back to thrust your hips forwards to an upright position. Contract your glutes at the top of the movement. Continue to repeat the exercise for the time given in your workout.

MAKE IT easier

If it is difficult to maintain balance, do the exercise without weights. Place your hands behind your head and extend your elbows out to the sides.

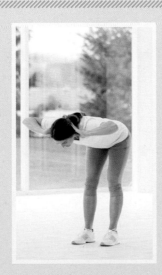

MAKE IT harder

To strengthen your upper back, after step 2, extend your arms straight down to lower the dumbbells. Then engage your upper-back muscles to pull the dumbbells back from your elbows before continuing to step 3.

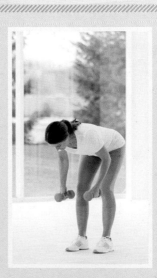

Sumo deadlift and upright row

IMPROVES
/// Posture
/// **Strength**
/// **Stability**
/// Mobility
/// **Endurance**

WHAT YOU NEED
Dumbbells

The deadlift is a full-body move that strengthens nearly every muscle in your body. Incorporating it with the wide stance enables you to more easily lift heavy objects. Perform this exercise to prevent or rehabilitate lifting injuries.

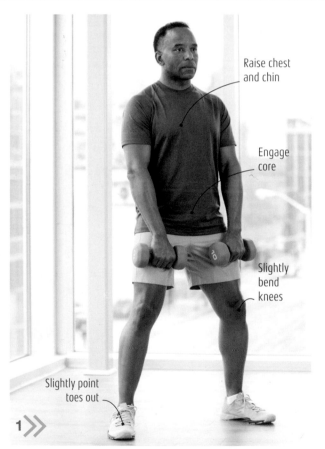

Raise chest and chin

Engage core

Slightly bend knees

Slightly point toes out

1 >>

Stand with your feet wider than shoulder-width apart. Hold a dumbbell in each hand, and let your arms hang in front of your body, palms facing your thighs. Engage your core and retract your shoulder blades.

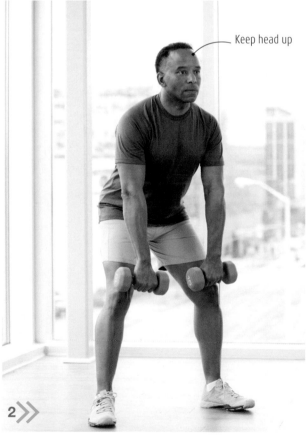

Keep head up

2 >>

Push your glutes back and bend at your hips, letting the dumbbells move downwards. Keep your back straight and hold your head up. Continue to retract your shoulder blades.

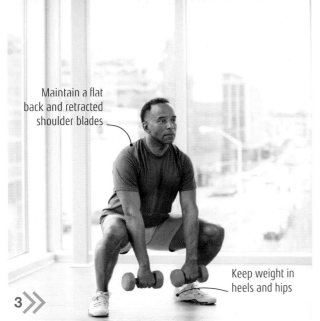

Maintain a flat back and retracted shoulder blades

Keep weight in heels and hips

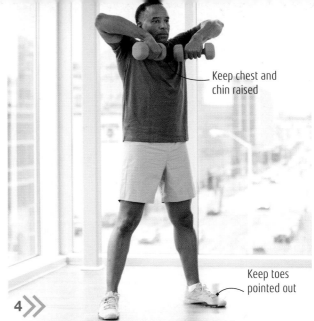

Keep chest and chin raised

Keep toes pointed out

3 » In a quick, controlled manner, continue to bend your knees and sit back into a squat until your thighs are parallel to the ground. Let the dumbbells hang straight down between your legs.

4 » In one swift motion, push through your heels and rise out of the squat until your legs are straight, and pull the dumbbells straight up until they are at chest height. Keep your core engaged.

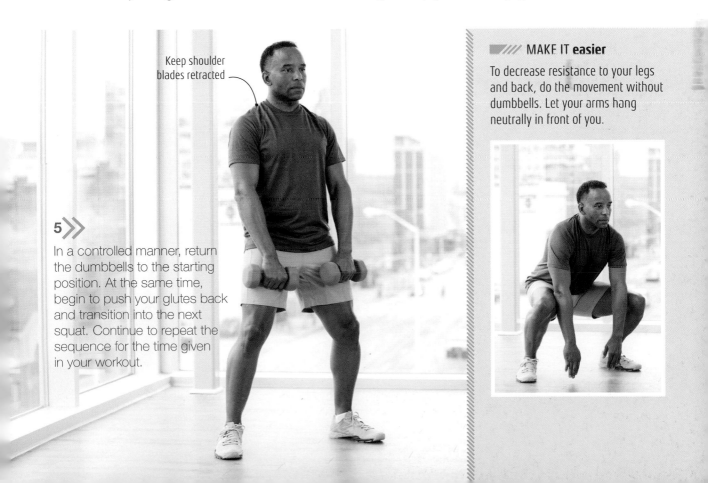

Keep shoulder blades retracted

5 » In a controlled manner, return the dumbbells to the starting position. At the same time, begin to push your glutes back and transition into the next squat. Continue to repeat the sequence for the time given in your workout.

/// MAKE IT **easier**

To decrease resistance to your legs and back, do the movement without dumbbells. Let your arms hang neutrally in front of you.

IMPROVES

///// Posture

///// **Strength**

///// **Stability**

///// Mobility

WHAT YOU NEED
Mat

Hip-ups

Your glutes can become weak and stiff when you don't use them often. Perform this powerful and controlled exercise to awaken your glutes and hip muscles and to improve your core and lower-body strength. This exercise will help you more safely execute common movements, such as standing up from a seated position.

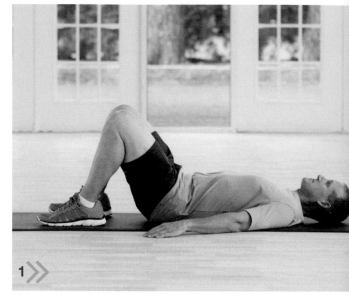

1 »

Lie on your back, bend your knees, and plant your feet flat on the ground, hip-width apart. Raise your chin and relax your arms by your sides, palms facing down.

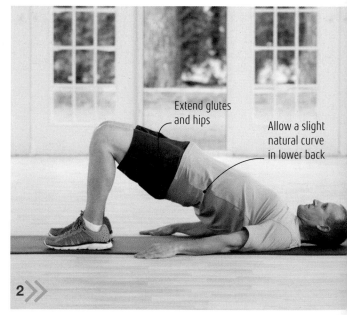

Extend glutes and hips

Allow a slight natural curve in lower back

2 »

Forcefully push your heels into the ground and raise your hips until you form a straight line from your knees to your shoulders. Contract your glutes and abdominals at the top of the movement.

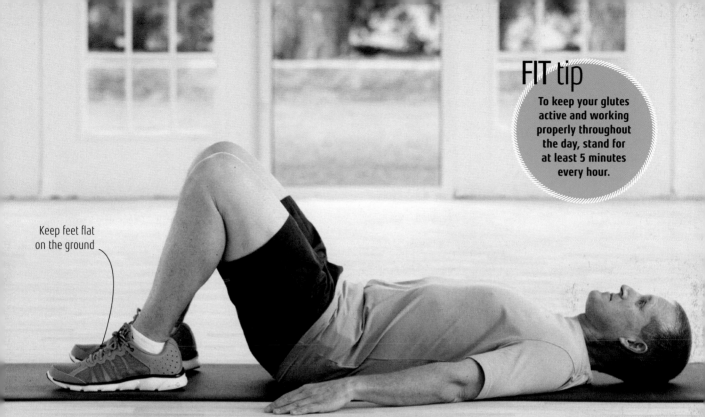

Keep feet flat on the ground

FIT tip

To keep your glutes active and working properly throughout the day, stand for at least 5 minutes every hour.

3 »

Using your glutes and abdominals for control, take three seconds to lower your hips to the ground. Continue to repeat the exercise for the time given in your workout.

///// MAKE IT harder

To increase resistance to your glutes, in step 2, raise one leg straight up until perpendicular to the ground. Push through your opposite heel to raise your hips. Then continue to step 3 while leaving your leg extended. Halfway through the given time, swap your legs.

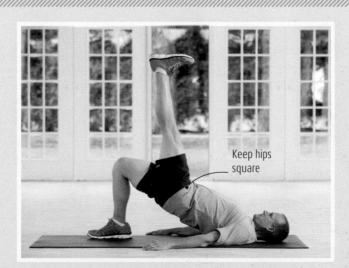

Keep hips square

Earthquakes

Many activities, such as digging with a spade, hammering, or pressing the lid down on a container, require you to generate downward power. Perform this total-body exercise swiftly to help you generate core strength for executing movements in a downward direction.

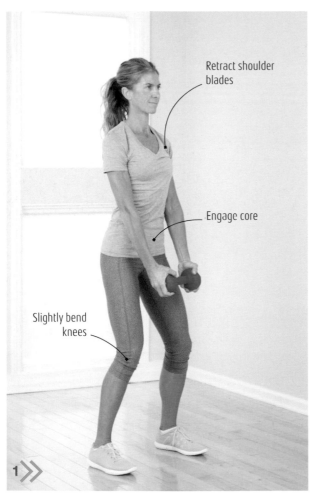

Retract shoulder blades

Engage core

Slightly bend knees

1 》》

Stand with your feet slightly wider than shoulder-width apart. Hold the ends of a dumbbell with both hands and let your arms hang straight down in front of you.

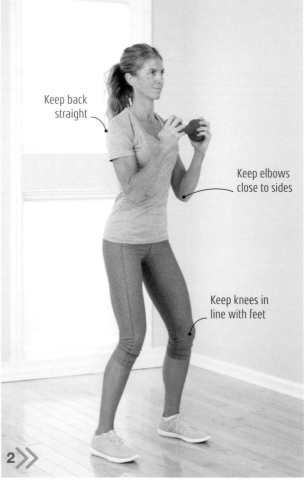

Keep back straight

Keep elbows close to sides

Keep knees in line with feet

2 》》

Engage your biceps to curl the dumbbell to chest height. Raise it through your elbows, which act as hinges. Continue to retract your shoulder blades.

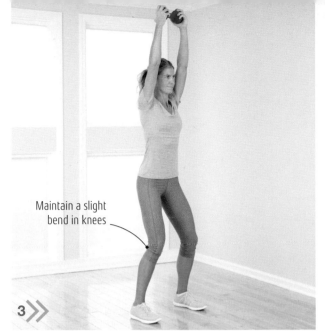

Maintain a slight
bend in knees

3 »

Engage your shoulders and triceps to press the
dumbbell straight up. Keep your elbows directly
under the dumbbell and keep your chin raised.

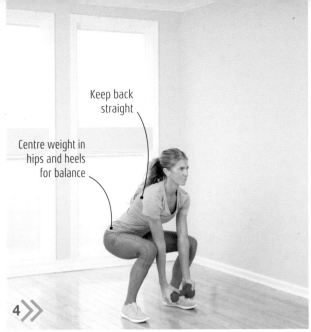

Keep back
straight

Centre weight in
hips and heels
for balance

4 »

In a continuous motion, sit your glutes back into a
squat until your thighs are parallel to the ground, and
powerfully thrust the dumbbell between your legs.

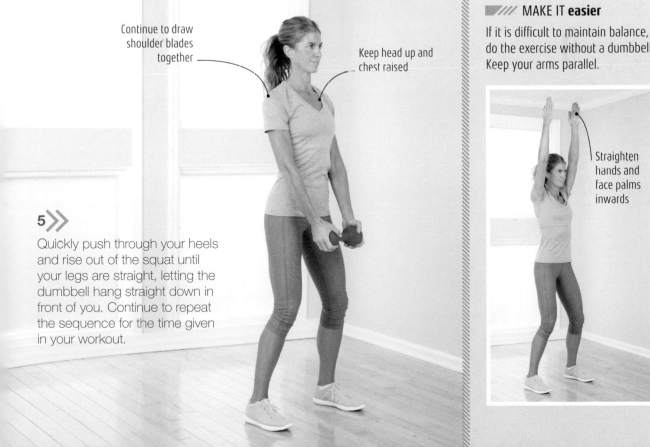

Continue to draw
shoulder blades
together

Keep head up and
chest raised

5 »

Quickly push through your heels
and rise out of the squat until
your legs are straight, letting the
dumbbell hang straight down in
front of you. Continue to repeat
the sequence for the time given
in your workout.

/// MAKE IT easier

If it is difficult to maintain balance,
do the exercise without a dumbbell.
Keep your arms parallel.

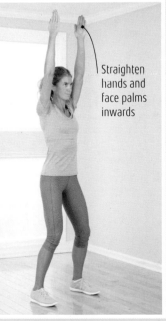

Straighten
hands and
face palms
inwards

IMPROVES
■//// **Strength**
■//// **Stability**
//// **Mobility**
■//// **Endurance**

WHAT YOU NEED
Step

Lateral step-ups

Many daily activities, such as climbing stairs, require your legs to work and balance independently. Build dexterity with this brisk stepping exercise that develops leg strength, improves stability, and resolves lower-body muscle imbalances.

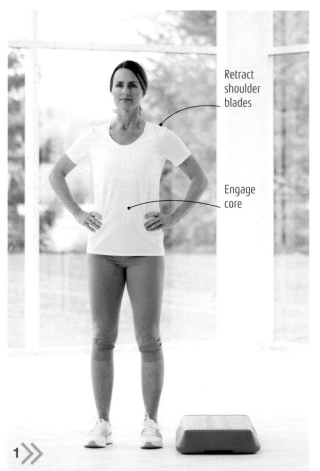

Retract shoulder blades

Engage core

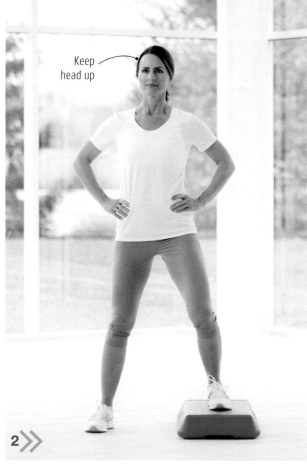

Keep head up

1 》

Stand to the right of a step or stair with your feet shoulder-width apart. Place your hands on your hips and slightly bend your knees. Engage your core and retract your shoulder blades.

2 》

Lift your left leg from the knee until your left foot is about 5cm (2in) above the step, then place your left foot fully on the step. Keep your torso upright and your chin raised.

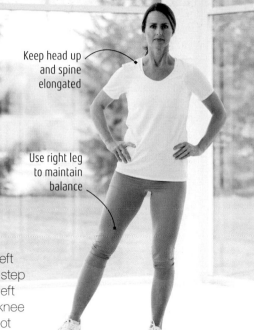

Keep head up and spine elongated

Use right leg to maintain balance

3 »

Shift your weight to your left foot and stand up on the step by pushing through your left heel and extending your knee and hips. Let your right foot come off the ground. Hold for one second.

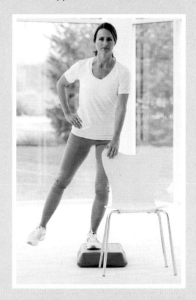

■//// MAKE IT **easier**

If it is difficult to maintain balance, lightly rest your hand on a chair or rail for support.

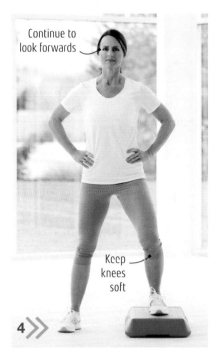

Continue to look forwards

Keep knees soft

4 »

Shift your weight back onto your right foot by lowering your right leg back to the ground. Slightly bend your knees and hips to absorb your weight.

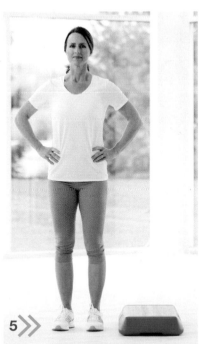

5 »

Return your left leg to the starting position. Repeat the exercise for the time given. Spend half the time stepping onto your left foot, then repeat on the opposite side.

■//// MAKE IT **harder**

To increase resistance to your legs, raise the height of the step.

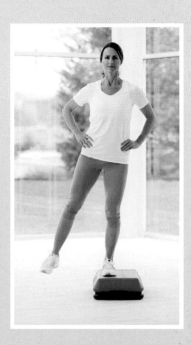

Overhead squat

Good mobility is a crucial aspect of staying fit, and it decreases your chance of injury while keeping your joints healthy. Perform this full-body squat to improve the range-of-motion of your ankles, knees, hips, back, and shoulders, while strengthening your legs.

IMPROVES
/// **Posture**
/// **Strength**
/// **Stability**
/// **Mobility**
/// **Endurance**

WHAT YOU NEED
No equipment needed

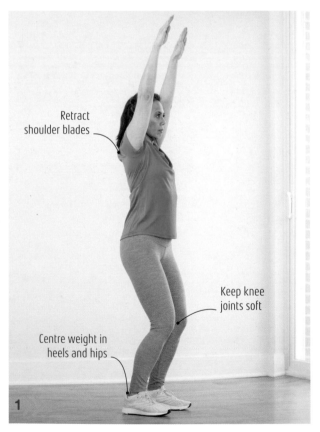

Retract shoulder blades

Keep knee joints soft

Centre weight in heels and hips

1

Stand with your feet shoulder-width apart. Raise both arms straight overhead at shoulder-width, fingers together and palms facing forwards. Engage your core and slightly bend your knees.

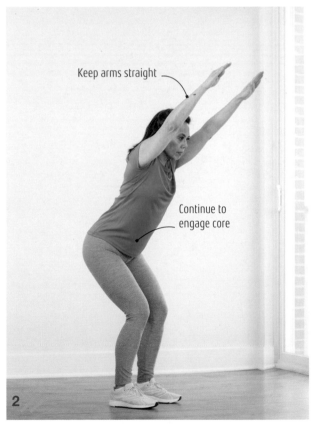

Keep arms straight

Continue to engage core

2

Push your glutes back and bend at your hips, keeping your arms aligned with your head. Keep your back straight and your toes pointed forwards. Keep your head raised.

3 »

In a quick, controlled manner, bend your knees to sit back into a squat until your thighs are parallel to the ground. Keep your body as upright as possible and avoid bending forwards at the waist. Distribute your weight in your hips and heels.

Pull arms back so they are in line with torso

Maintain a straight line from hips to hands

Keep feet flat on the ground

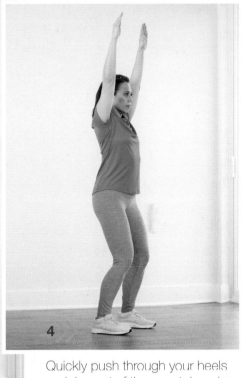

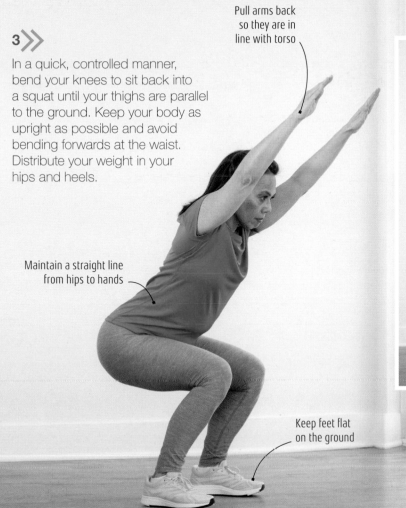

4

Quickly push through your heels and rise out of the squat, keeping your shoulder blades retracted and your back straight. Continue to repeat the exercise for the time given in your workout.

///// MAKE IT **easier**

If you have limited flexibility, place a folded mat under your heels to elevate them about 5cm (2in) while you perform the squat.

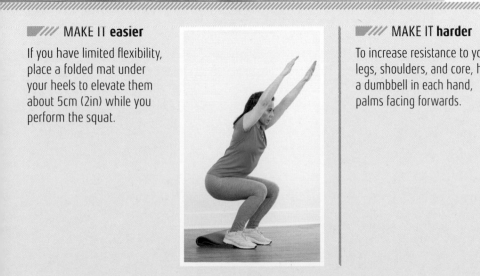

///// MAKE IT **harder**

To increase resistance to your legs, shoulders, and core, hold a dumbbell in each hand, palms facing forwards.

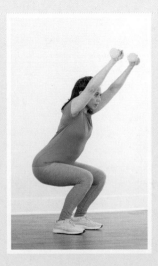

IMPROVES

//// Posture

//// **Strength**

//// **Stability**

//// Mobility

//// **Endurance**

WHAT YOU NEED
Dumbbells

Stationary lunge and curl

Lunges not only strengthen your legs, but they also do a remarkable job of stretching your hips. Perform this exercise for strong and flexible hip flexors, which are essential for preventing hip, knee, and lower-back pain.

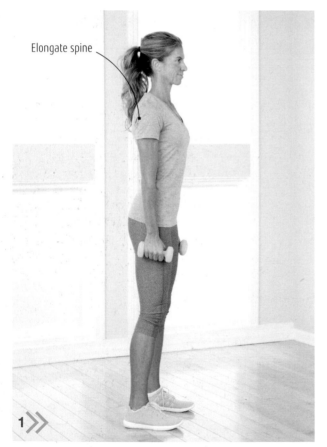

Elongate spine

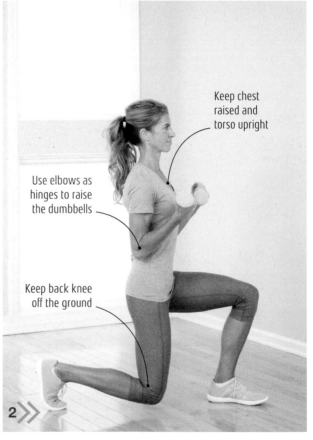

Keep chest raised and torso upright

Use elbows as hinges to raise the dumbbells

Keep back knee off the ground

1 >>
Stand with your feet shoulder-width apart. Hold a dumbbell in each hand, palms facing inwards, and let your arms hang at your sides. Engage your core and retract your shoulder blades. Raise your chin.

2 >>
In one quick, controlled motion, take a long step forwards with your left leg, drop your right knee down until both knees are bent to 90 degrees, and curl the dumbbells to chest height, palms facing towards you.

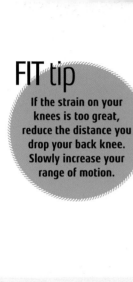

FIT tip

If the strain on your knees is too great, reduce the distance you drop your back knee. Slowly increase your range of motion.

Continue to draw shoulder blades together

Rotate palms back towards body

3 »

Quickly engage both legs to return to the starting position, while using your biceps to lower the dumbbells and rotate your arms back to the starting position. Repeat the lunge by stepping forwards with your right leg. Alternate lunging on each side for the time given in your workout.

MAKE IT **easier**

To decrease resistance to your legs, in step 1, step your right leg back into a staggered stance. In step 2, drop your right knee into a lunge. Then exit the lunge, but remain in the staggered stance. Reverse your stance halfway through.

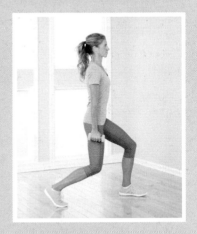

MAKE IT **harder**

To strengthen your shoulders, after step 2, rotate your hands 180 degrees and press the dumbbells straight overhead, then return the dumbbells to the top of the curl position. Continue to step 3.

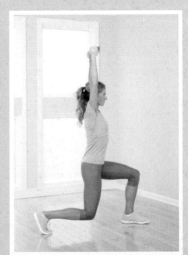

Side lunge

The human body is not only designed to move forwards and backwards – but also from side to side. Perform this exercise in a quick and controlled manner to strengthen your hip adductors and glutes so you can cope better with the stresses of lateral movement.

IMPROVES
/// Strength
/// Stability
/// Mobility
/// Endurance

WHAT YOU NEED
No equipment needed

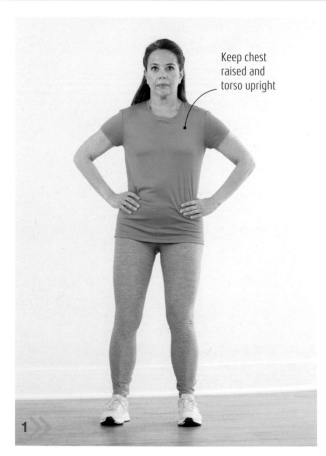

Keep chest raised and torso upright

1

Stand with your feet shoulder-width apart and place your hands on your hips. Slightly bend your knees. Engage your core and retract your shoulder blades.

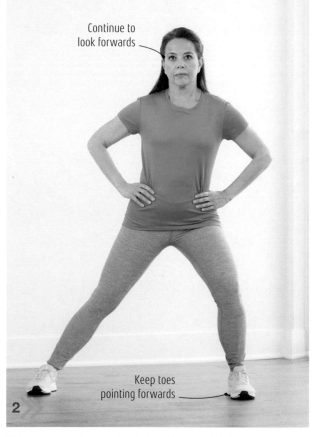

Continue to look forwards

Keep toes pointing forwards

2

Take a long step to the left with your left leg, landing first on the heel of your foot, and slightly bend your left knee. Keep your right leg straight.

3 »

Continue to bend your left knee, push your glutes back, and bend at the hips until your left thigh is parallel to the ground.

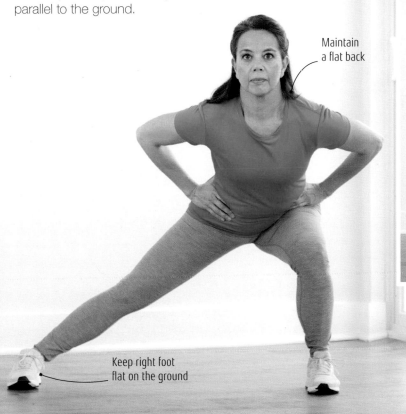

Maintain a flat back

Keep right foot flat on the ground

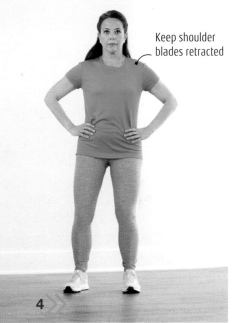

Keep shoulder blades retracted

4 »

Push through your left heel and engage your legs to return to the starting position. Repeat the exercise to your right. Alternate lunging to each side for the time given in your workout.

///// MAKE IT **easier**

To decrease the load on your legs, in step 2, take a shorter step out with your left leg. In step 3, push your glutes back until your thighs are parallel to the ground. In step 4, push through your left heel to stand up and step your leg back to the starting position. Repeat with your right leg.

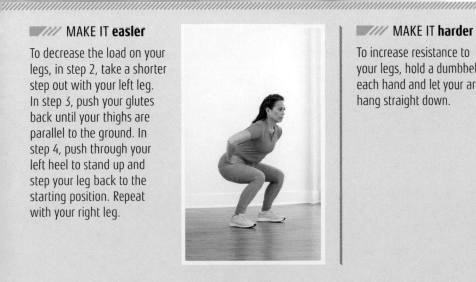

///// MAKE IT **harder**

To increase resistance to your legs, hold a dumbbell in each hand and let your arms hang straight down.

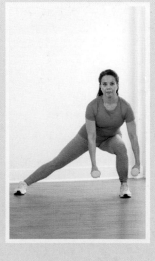

IMPROVES

/// Posture

/// **Strength**

/// **Stability**

/// Mobility

/// **Endurance**

WHAT YOU NEED
Dumbbells

Split squat and thruster

A principle of functional training is to choose movements that work multiple body parts together. This efficient squat and upper-body exercise uses several muscle chains at once. Perform it in a swift manner to strengthen your quadriceps, calves, glutes, lower back, hamstrings, triceps, and shoulders.

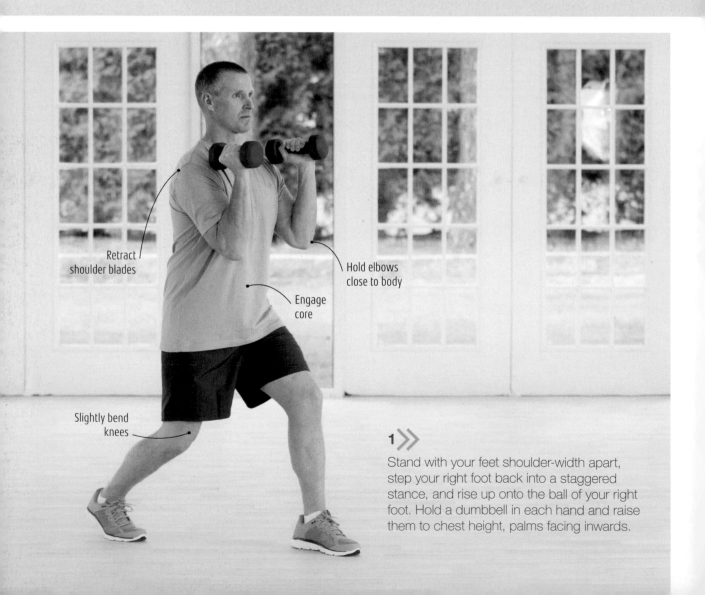

Retract shoulder blades

Hold elbows close to body

Engage core

Slightly bend knees

1 »

Stand with your feet shoulder-width apart, step your right foot back into a staggered stance, and rise up onto the ball of your right foot. Hold a dumbbell in each hand and raise them to chest height, palms facing inwards.

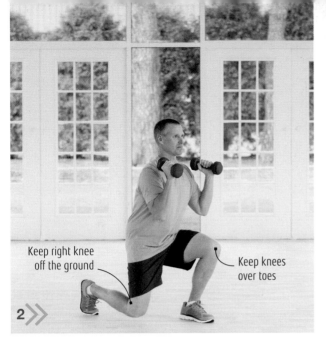

Keep right knee
off the ground

Keep knees
over toes

2 ≫

Keeping your arms in position, drop your right knee straight down until both knees are bent to 90 degrees. Keep your back straight and your head raised.

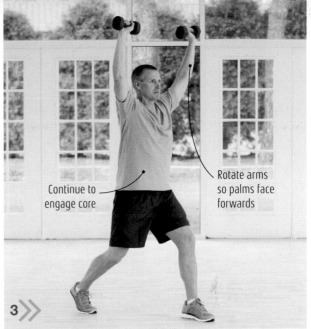

Continue to
engage core

Rotate arms
so palms face
forwards

3 ≫

In one swift motion, engage both legs to return to the staggered stance, rotate your arms 90 degrees forwards, and press the dumbbells overhead.

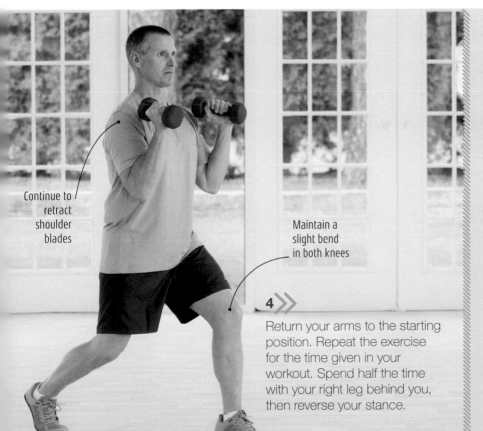

Continue to
retract
shoulder
blades

Maintain a
slight bend
in both knees

4 ≫

Return your arms to the starting position. Repeat the exercise for the time given in your workout. Spend half the time with your right leg behind you, then reverse your stance.

///// MAKE IT easier

If it is difficult to maintain balance, in step 1, stand with your feet shoulder-width apart. In step 2, squat until your thighs are parallel to the ground. In step 3, stand up by pushing through your heels.

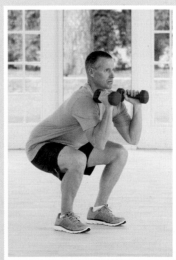

WORKOUT
ROUTINES

Don't just work hard – work smart. These workout routines are collections of exercises purposefully designed to help you achieve your fitness goals. Complete the routines as required by your programme to ensure that the time you spend training works your body in a safe, healthy, and balanced way.

Warm up

Dynamic stretches prepare your body for a good workout by increasing your blood flow and muscle temperature. Follow this method before every workout to improve your range of motion, activate your muscles, and prevent injury.

WHAT YOU NEED

No equipment needed

YOUR WORKOUT

- Before every workout, perform the entire sequence of warm-up exercises in order two times. Use a stopwatch to follow the work and rest intervals.
- Do not use dumbbells for any of these exercises.
- Focus on your goals and mentally prepare yourself to work hard.

THE LEVELS

ALL LEVELS

Carry out the exercise sequence
2 times

Perform each exercise for
20 seconds

Rest between each exercise for
10 seconds

Total time
5 minutes

THE EXERCISES

1	HIGH KNEE AND REACH	p.34
2	STANDING TWIST	p.108
3	POSTERIOR SWING	p.130
4	ARM PULLOVERS	p.78
5	OVERHEAD SQUAT	p.142

5-minute kick-start

Just 5 minutes of activity a day is enough to reduce your chance of heart disease by 45 per cent. Use this efficient, total-body workout whenever you are running short of time and want a quick boost of energy that is good for your whole body.

WHAT YOU NEED
Dumbbells, table top, mat

YOUR WORKOUT
- Select the level as required by your exercise programme.
- Perform the entire sequence of exercises in order one time. Use a stopwatch to follow the work and rest intervals.
- If it is difficult to balance, try an easier modification or reduce the weight of your dumbbells.

THE LEVELS

LEVEL 1

Carry out the exercise sequence **1 time**

Perform each exercise for **20 seconds**

Rest between each exercise for **10 seconds**

Total time **5 minutes**

LEVEL 2

Carry out the exercise sequence **1 time**

Perform each exercise for **25 seconds**

Rest between each exercise for **5 seconds**

Total time **5 minutes**

LEVEL 3

Carry out the exercise sequence **1 time**

Perform each exercise for **30 seconds**

Rest between each exercise for **0 seconds**

Total time **5 minutes**

THE EXERCISES

1	HIGH KNEE AND REACH	p.34
2	INCLINED PUSH-UPS	p.54
3	HIP-UPS	p.136
4	FAST FEET	p.26
5	SUITCASE ROW	p.72
6	SUITCASE SQUAT	p.124
7	KNEE CHOP	p.104
8	PUSH PRESS	p.60
9	SPLIT STANCE RUNNERS	p.100
10	SUMO DEADLIFT AND UPRIGHT ROW	p.134

Cardiovascular endurance

Consistent cardiovascular exercise helps you live longer and improves your heart health and quality of life. Perform this routine vigorously to strengthen your heart, increase lung capacity, support better sleep, and improve energy levels.

WHAT YOU NEED

Dumbbells, step, chair

YOUR WORKOUT

- Select the level as required by your exercise programme.
- Perform the entire sequence of exercises in order for the prescribed number of times. Use a stopwatch to follow the work and rest intervals.
- Exert maximum aerobic effort, and use the rest times between each exercise to gear up for the next drill.

THE LEVELS

LEVEL 1

Carry out the exercise sequence **2 times**

Perform each exercise for **20 seconds**

Rest between each exercise for **10 seconds**

Total time **10 minutes**

LEVEL 2

Carry out the exercise sequence **3 times**

Perform each exercise for **30 seconds**

Rest between each exercise for **10 seconds**

Total time **20 minutes**

LEVEL 3

Carry out the exercise sequence **3 times**

Perform each exercise for **35 seconds**

Rest between each exercise for **5 seconds**

Total time **20 minutes**

THE EXERCISES

1	SIDE SHUFFLE	p.30
2	SIDE-TO-SIDE PUNCH	p.106
3	STEP-UPS	p.40
4	ARM PULLOVERS	p.78
5	FAUX SKIPPING	p.44
6	WOOD CHOP	p.102
7	CHAIR MOUNTAIN CLIMBER	p.46
8	ONE-ARM LIFT	p.86
9	SWITCH JUMPS	p.48
10	CURL AND SHOULDER PRESS AND REACH	p.56

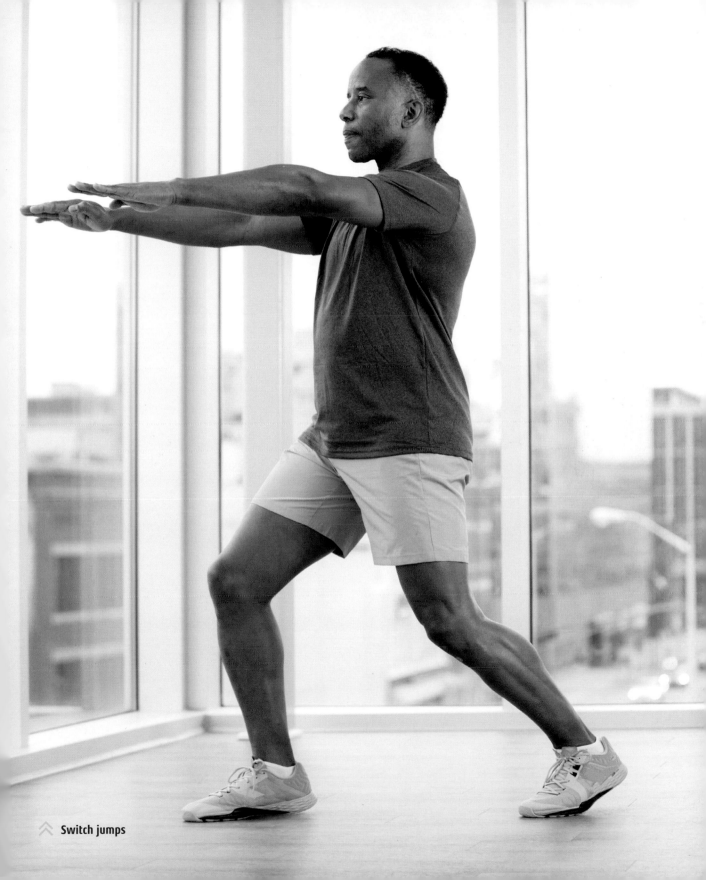

Switch jumps

Beginner total body

Limited mobility does not mean you cannot exercise. If you are new to exercise, recovering from an injury, or have trouble balancing, this routine uses the seated versions of exercises to help you gain strength and improve cardiovascular endurance.

WHAT YOU NEED
Dumbbells, chair

YOUR WORKOUT

- Select the level as required by your exercise programme.
- Perform the entire sequence of exercises in order two times. Use a stopwatch to follow the work and rest intervals.
- Do the seated modification for each exercise.

THE LEVELS

LEVEL 1

Carry out the exercise sequence
2 times

Perform each exercise for
15 seconds

Rest between each exercise for
15 seconds

Total time
9 minutes

LEVEL 2

Carry out the exercise sequence
2 times

Perform each exercise for
20 seconds

Rest between each exercise for
10 seconds

Total time
9 minutes

LEVEL 3

Carry out the exercise sequence
2 times

Perform each exercise for
30 seconds

Rest between each exercise for
10 seconds

Total time
12 minutes

THE EXERCISES

1	MARCH IN PLACE	p.32
2	BENT ROW AND HAMMER CURL	p.82
3	PUSH PRESS	p.60
4	FAST FEET	p.26
5	STAGGERED REVERSE FLY	p.76
6	GUNSLINGER	p.68
7	HIGH KNEE AND REACH	p.34
8	SEESAW ROW	p.94
9	ONE-ARM MILITARY PRESS	p.50

Low-intensity strength

It is never too late to start building muscle mass. Adding strength training to your programme is one of the best ways to prevent or reverse bone loss and muscle atrophy. Perform these exercises to ease your way safely into resistance training.

WHAT YOU NEED
Dumbbells, table top

YOUR WORKOUT

- Select the level as required by your exercise programme.
- Perform the entire sequence of exercises in order for the prescribed number of times. Use a stopwatch to follow the work and rest intervals.
- It is okay to start without dumbbells. You can slowly increase your resistance each time you perform the routine.

THE LEVELS

LEVEL 1

Carry out the exercise sequence
2 times

Perform each exercise for
20 seconds

Rest between each exercise for
10 seconds

Total time
10 minutes

LEVEL 2

Carry out the exercise sequence
2 times

Perform each exercise for
30 seconds

Rest between each exercise for
10 seconds

Total time
13 minutes

LEVEL 3

Carry out the exercise sequence
3 times

Perform each exercise for
30 seconds

Rest between each exercise for
10 seconds

Total time
20 minutes

THE EXERCISES

1	ONE-ARM CHEST PRESS	p.62
2	SUITCASE ROW	p.72
3	SUITCASE SQUAT	p.124
4	STANDING TWIST	p.108
5	PUSH PRESS	p.60
6	SUMO DEADLIFT AND UPRIGHT ROW	p.134
7	CURL FROM ONE LEG	p.96
8	INCLINED PUSH-UPS	p.54
9	WALKING REACHING LUNGE	p.126
10	WINDMILL	p.118

Speed and agility

Athleticism requires a combination of speed, agility, reaction time, and power. For non-athletes and weekend warriors alike, this routine will enhance athletic ability with power drills that improve footwork and boost total-body coordination.

WHAT YOU NEED
Dumbbells, chair, table top

YOUR WORKOUT
- Select your level according to your workout programme.
- Perform the entire sequence of exercises in order for the prescribed number of times. Use a stopwatch to follow the work and rest intervals.
- Begin your workout with no weights or with light dumbbells, and increase resistance as you are able.

THE LEVELS

LEVEL 1

Carry out the exercise sequence
2 times

Perform each exercise for
15 seconds

Rest between each exercise for
15 seconds

Total time
10 minutes

LEVEL 2

Carry out the exercise sequence
3 times

Perform each exercise for
30 seconds

Rest between each exercise for
15 seconds

Total time
22 minutes

LEVEL 3

Carry out the exercise sequence
3 times

Perform each exercise for
40 seconds

Rest between each exercise for
10 seconds

Total time
25 minutes

THE EXERCISES

1	CHAIR MOUNTAIN CLIMBER	p.46
2	SHOT-PUT PRESS	p.70
3	SIDE LUNGE	p.146
4	LAWN MOWER ROW	p.74
5	CROSS-COUNTRY SKIERS	p.42
6	INCLINED PUSH-UPS	p.54
7	SPLIT STANCE RUNNERS	p.100
8	REVERSE LUNGE WITH TWIST	p.128
9	EARTHQUAKES	p.138
10	SEESAW ROW	p.94

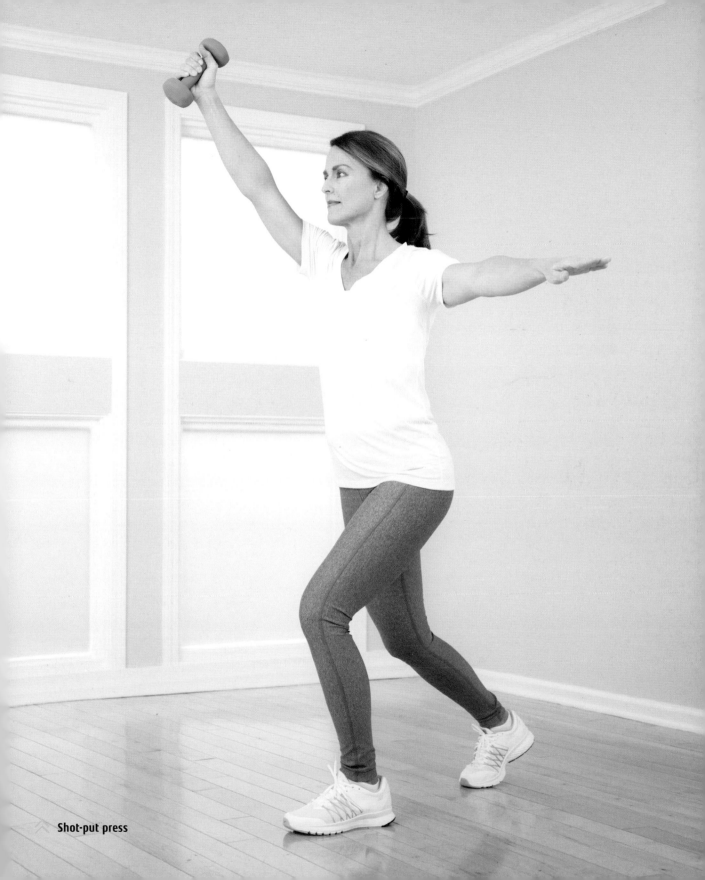

Shot-put press

Balance and stability

Control of your core and the muscles that surround your ankles, knees, hips, and shoulders is essential for good balance. Follow this routine to train those muscles, improve your posture, enhance your coordination, and boost your stability.

WHAT YOU NEED
Dumbbells, step

YOUR WORKOUT
- Select the level as required by your exercise programme.
- Perform the entire sequence of exercises in order two times. Use a stopwatch to follow the work and rest intervals.
- If it is difficult to balance, try an easier modification or reduce the weight of your dumbbells.

THE LEVELS

LEVEL 1

Carry out the exercise sequence
2 times

Perform each exercise for
15 seconds

Rest between each exercise for
15 seconds

Total time
10 minutes

LEVEL 2

Carry out the exercise sequence
2 times

Perform each exercise for
20 seconds

Rest between each exercise for
10 seconds

Total time
10 minutes

LEVEL 3

Carry out the exercise sequence
2 times

Perform each exercise for
30 seconds

Rest between each exercise for
10 seconds

Total time
13 minutes

THE EXERCISES

1	HIGH KNEE AND REACH	p.34
2	CURL FROM ONE LEG	p.96
3	REVERSE LUNGE WITH TWIST	p.128
4	SUITCASE ROW	p.72
5	LATERAL STEP-UPS	p.140
6	CROSSOVER TOE TOUCH	p.114
7	ONE-LEG ARM RAISE	p.64
8	SUITCASE SQUAT	p.124
9	STANDING ELBOW TO KNEE	p.98
10	ONE-ARM MILITARY PRESS	p.50

Total-body mobility

Mobility is your body's ability to move freely without undue stress. Perform the exercises in this routine to increase the range of motion in your muscles and joints, improve your flexibility, and decrease strain on your body's systems.

WHAT YOU NEED
Dumbbells, chair, wall

YOUR WORKOUT

- Select the level as required by your exercise programme.
- Perform the entire sequence of exercises in order two times. Use a stopwatch to follow the work and rest intervals.
- If any movements are painful, immediately try the modification or skip the exercise until your mobility improves.

THE LEVELS

LEVEL 1

Carry out the exercise sequence
2 times

Perform each exercise for
15 seconds

Rest between each exercise for
15 seconds

Total time
10 minutes

LEVEL 2

Carry out the exercise sequence
2 times

Perform each exercise for
20 seconds

Rest between each exercise for
10 seconds

Total time
10 minutes

LEVEL 3

Carry out the exercise sequence
2 times

Perform each exercise for
30 seconds

Rest between each exercise for
10 seconds

Total time
13 minutes

THE EXERCISES

1	GOOD MORNING	p.132
2	SIDE-TO-SIDE PUNCH	p.106
3	OVERHEAD SQUAT	p.142
4	ARM PULLOVERS	p.78
5	CHEST OPENER	p.58
6	REVERSE LUNGE WITH TWIST	p.128
7	WINDMILL	p.118
8	CHAIR DIPS	p.52
9	KNEE CHOP	p.104
10	WALL ANGEL	p.84

Cross-training

To advance your fitness level, it's necessary to keep your body alert by including variety in your workouts. This cross-training routine combines strength, aerobic, and flexibility exercises to challenge your body and help you avoid fitness plateaus.

WHAT YOU NEED
Dumbbells, mat, step

YOUR WORKOUT
- Select the level as required by your exercise programme.
- Perform the entire sequence of exercises in order for the prescribed number of times. Use a stopwatch to follow the work and rest intervals.
- If you are unable to complete a round of the sequence, reduce the weight of your dumbbells or choose an easier modification.

THE LEVELS

LEVEL 1

Carry out the exercise sequence **2 times**

Perform each exercise for **15 seconds**

Rest between each exercise for **15 seconds**

Total time **10 minutes**

LEVEL 2

Carry out the exercise sequence **3 times**

Perform each exercise for **30 seconds**

Rest between each exercise for **15 seconds**

Total time **22 minutes**

LEVEL 3

Carry out the exercise sequence **3 times**

Perform each exercise for **40 seconds**

Rest between each exercise for **10 seconds**

Total time **25 minutes**

THE EXERCISES

1	HIGH PLANK ROW	p.90
2	OVER-THE-SHOULDER SQUAT	p.120
3	FARMER'S WALK	p.36
4	ONE-LEG ARM RAISE	p.64
5	POSTERIOR SWING	p.130
6	SPLIT SQUAT AND THRUSTER	p.148
7	WINDMILL	p.118
8	LATERAL STEP-UPS	p.140
9	STAGGERED REVERSE FLY	p.76
10	SIDE SHUFFLE	p.30

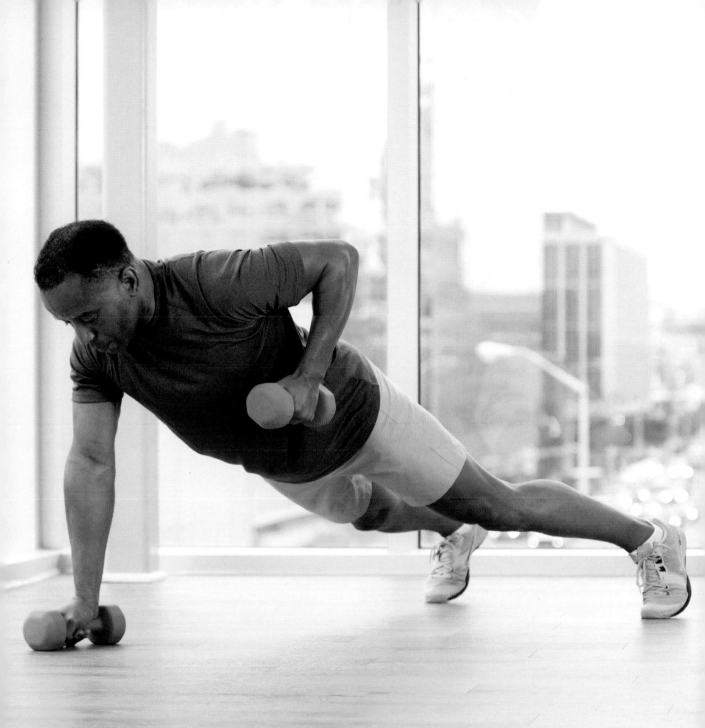

High plank row

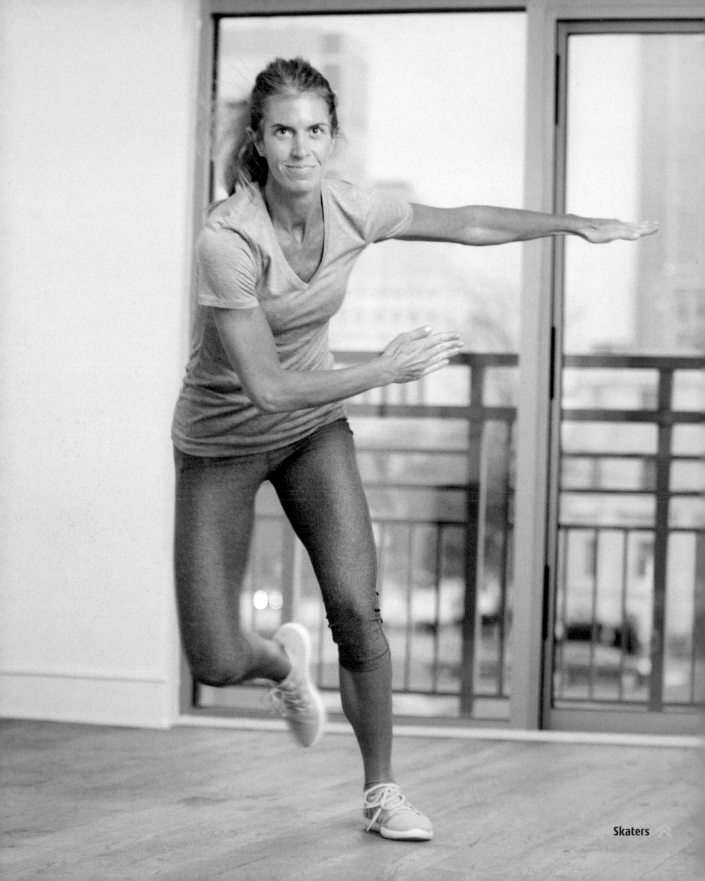

Skaters

Calorie-burning HIIT

High-intensity interval training (HIIT) is a method of exercise that alternates short bursts of intense exercise and short periods of rest. Work as hard and quickly as you can during this routine to burn a high volume of calories and fat in a short time.

WHAT YOU NEED
Dumbbells, mat, step, chair

YOUR WORKOUT

- Select the level as required by your exercise programme.
- Perform the entire sequence of exercises in order for the prescribed number of times. Use a stopwatch to follow the work and rest intervals.
- Maintain a steady breathing pattern — in through your nose and out through your mouth — so you have the necessary oxygen to generate energy.

THE LEVELS

LEVEL 1

Carry out the exercise sequence
2 times

Perform each exercise for
15 seconds

Rest between each exercise for
15 seconds

Total time
10 minutes

LEVEL 2

Carry out the exercise sequence
3 times

Perform each exercise for
30 seconds

Rest between each exercise for
10 seconds

Total time
20 minutes

LEVEL 3

Carry out the exercise sequence
3 times

Perform each exercise for
40 seconds

Rest between each exercise for
10 seconds

Total time
25 minutes

THE EXERCISES

1	SUMO DEADLIFT AND UPRIGHT ROW	p.134
2	SKATERS	p.38
3	GUNSLINGER	p.68
4	HIGH PLANK REACH-THROUGH AND FLY	p.116
5	DIAGONAL CHOP	p.122
6	STEP-UPS	p.40
7	CHAIR DIPS	p.52
8	ROTATIONAL GOBLET SQUAT	p.112
9	BENT ROW AND HAMMER CURL	p.82
10	FAUX SKIPPING	p.44

Prehabilitation

One injury can stay with you for the rest of your life. Be proactive and use the *prehabilitation* method to help prevent injuries before they happen. These exercises will target and strengthen the areas of your body that are most susceptible to damage.

WHAT YOU NEED
Dumbbells, mat, wall, step

YOUR WORKOUT

- Select the level as required by your exercise programme.
- Perform the entire sequence of exercises in order for the prescribed number of times. Use a stopwatch to follow the work and rest intervals.
- Prioritize proper technique for each exercise rather than speed, and focus on using steady, controlled movements.

THE LEVELS

LEVEL 1

Carry out the exercise sequence
1 time

Perform each exercise for
20 seconds

Rest between each exercise for
15 seconds

Total time
**4 minutes
30 seconds**

LEVEL 2

Carry out the exercise sequence
2 times

Perform each exercise for
20 seconds

Rest between each exercise for
5 seconds

Total time
**6 minutes
30 seconds**

LEVEL 3

Carry out the exercise sequence
2 times

Perform each exercise for
30 seconds

Rest between each exercise for
5 seconds

Total time
9 minutes

THE EXERCISES

1	UPRIGHT EXTERNAL ROTATION	p.80
2	BIRD DOG	p.88
3	WALL ANGEL	p.84
4	STANDING TWIST	p.108
5	LATERAL STEP-UPS	p.140
6	CHEST OPENER	p.58
7	HIP-UPS	p.136
8	JUMPING WALL PUSH-UPS	p.66

Posture improvement

Prolonged sitting weakens your posture and wears out your muscles and joints, leading to discomfort in your neck, back, and hips. This routine strengthens those muscles so they support proper alignment and reduce the strain on your bones.

WHAT YOU NEED
Dumbbells, mat, wall

YOUR WORKOUT

- Select the level as required by your exercise programme.
- Perform the entire sequence of exercises in order for the prescribed number of times. Use a stopwatch to follow the work and rest intervals.
- Remember to breathe deeply during every movement so your muscles are receptive to stretching and strengthening.

THE LEVELS

LEVEL 1

Carry out the exercise sequence
2 times

Perform each exercise for
30 seconds

Rest between each exercise for
15 seconds

Total time
7 minutes

LEVEL 2

Carry out the exercise sequence
2 times

Perform each exercise for
30 seconds

Rest between each exercise for
10 seconds

Total time
**6 minutes
30 seconds**

LEVEL 3

Carry out the exercise sequence
3 times

Perform each exercise for
30 seconds

Rest between each exercise for
10 seconds

Total time
10 minutes

THE EXERCISES

1	STAGGERED REVERSE FLY	p.76
2	CHEST OPENER	p.58
3	REVERSE LUNGE WITH TWIST	p.128
4	BIRD DOG	p.88
5	WALL ANGEL	p.84

Core strength

Movements such as twisting, bending, and reaching require your lower back and abdominal muscles to work together. This routine includes rotational exercises to activate those muscles, improve your flexibility, and enhance your core stability.

WHAT YOU NEED
Dumbbells

YOUR WORKOUT

- Select the level as required by your exercise programme.
- Perform the entire sequence of exercises in order for the prescribed number of times. Use a stopwatch to follow the work and rest intervals.
- If any movements are too strenuous, reduce the weight of your dumbbells or try an easier modification.

THE LEVELS

LEVEL 1

Carry out the exercise sequence
1 time

Perform each exercise for
30 seconds

Rest between each exercise for
10 seconds

Total time
**6 minutes
30 seconds**

LEVEL 2

Carry out the exercise sequence
2 times

Perform each exercise for
30 seconds

Rest between each exercise for
10 seconds

Total time
13 minutes

LEVEL 3

Carry out the exercise sequence
3 times

Perform each exercise for
40 seconds

Rest between each exercise for
10 seconds

Total time
25 minutes

THE EXERCISES

1	STANDING ELBOW TO KNEE	p.98
2	WINDMILL	p.118
3	KNEE CHOP	p.104
4	STANDING OBLIQUE ROTATION	p.110
5	SIDE-TO-SIDE PUNCH	p.106
6	WOOD CHOP	p.102
7	CROSSOVER TOE TOUCH	p.114
8	DIAGONAL CHOP	p.122
9	STANDING TWIST	p.108
10	STANDING ELBOW TO KNEE	p.98

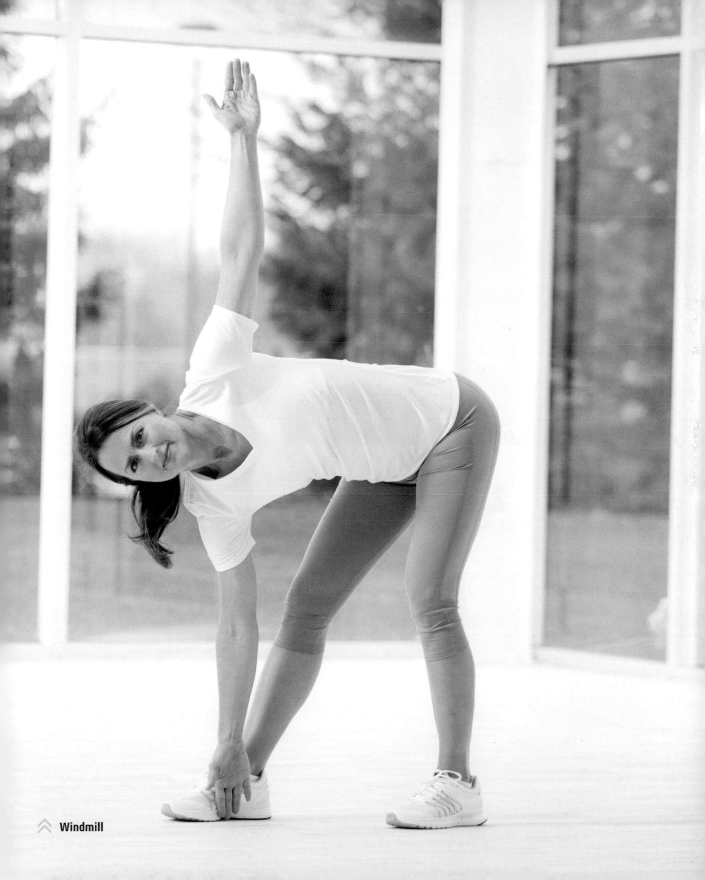

Windmill

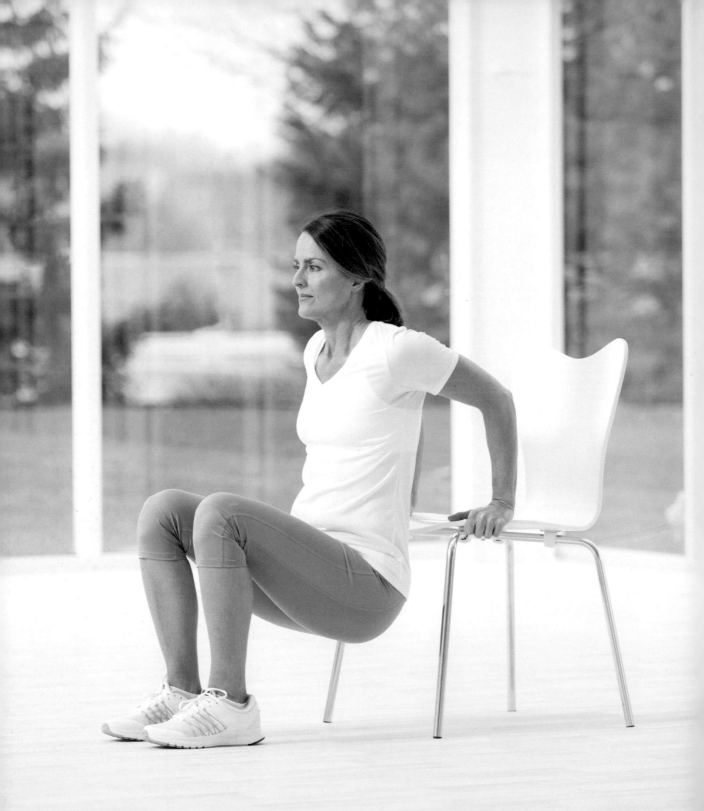

Chair dips

Total-body strength 1

Strength training tones and defines your muscles and makes your body more functional. The resistance exercises in this routine will protect your bones, aid weight loss, and build more lean muscle so your movements are safer and less strenuous.

WHAT YOU NEED
Dumbbells, chair, mat

YOUR WORKOUT

- Select the level as required by your exercise programme.
- Perform the entire sequence of exercises in order for the prescribed number of times. Use a stopwatch to follow the work and rest intervals.
- Use slow, controlled movements to maximize muscle recruitment and avoid relying on momentum to move yourself or the weights.

THE LEVELS

LEVEL 1

Carry out the exercise sequence
2 times

Perform each exercise for
20 seconds

Rest between each exercise for
10 seconds

Total time
10 minutes

LEVEL 2

Carry out the exercise sequence
3 times

Perform each exercise for
30 seconds

Rest between each exercise for
15 seconds

Total time
22 minutes

LEVEL 3

Carry out the exercise sequence
3 times

Perform each exercise for
40 seconds

Rest between each exercise for
10 seconds

Total time
25 minutes

THE EXERCISES

1	LAWN MOWER ROW	p.74
2	CHAIR DIPS	p.52
3	STANDING OBLIQUE ROTATION	p.110
4	STIFF-LEG DEADLIFT AND SHRUG	p.92
5	CURL AND SHOULDER PRESS AND REACH	p.56
6	SIDE LUNGE	p.146
7	FARMER'S WALK	p.36
8	HIGH PLANK REACH-THROUGH AND FLY	p.116
9	GUNSLINGER	p.68
10	ROTATIONAL GOBLET SQUAT	p.112

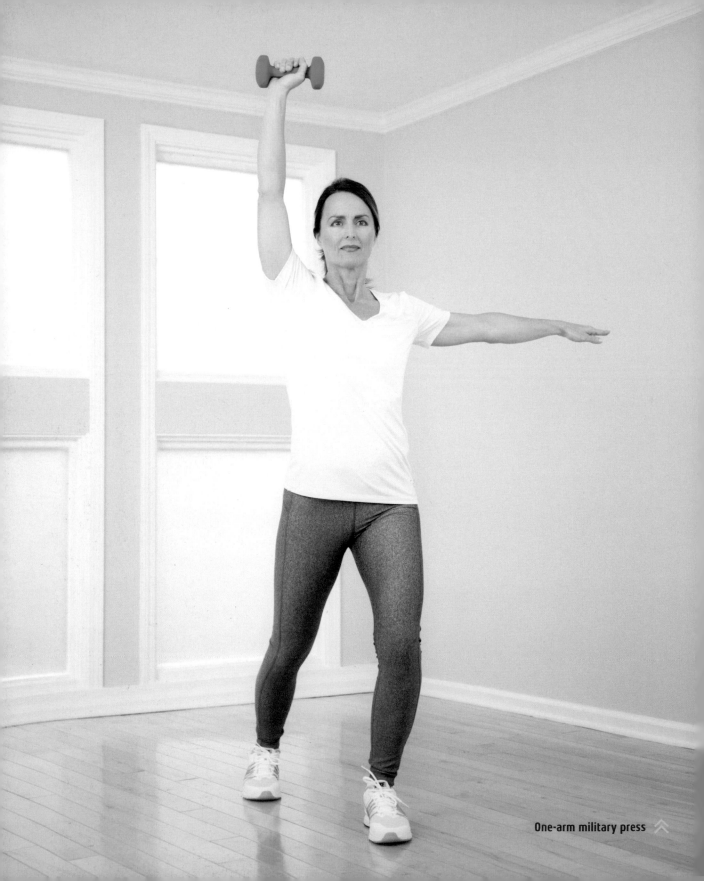

One-arm military press ⌃

Total-body strength 2

Do not underestimate the necessity of improving strength. With age, your metabolism can slow, your bones can weaken, and your posture can slump. Build muscle tissue with these exercises to offset the ageing process.

WHAT YOU NEED
Dumbbells, chair

YOUR WORKOUT

- Select the level as required by your exercise programme.
- Perform the entire sequence of exercises in order for the prescribed number of times. Use a stopwatch to follow the work and rest intervals.
- If you cannot maintain proper form or fully execute a movement, then reduce your resistance or don't use weights at all.

THE LEVELS

LEVEL 1

Carry out the exercise sequence **2 times**

Perform each exercise for **20 seconds**

Rest between each exercise for **10 seconds**

Total time **10 minutes**

LEVEL 2

Carry out the exercise sequence **3 times**

Perform each exercise for **30 seconds**

Rest between each exercise for **15 seconds**

Total time **22 minutes**

LEVEL 3

Carry out the exercise sequence **3 times**

Perform each exercise for **40 seconds**

Rest between each exercise for **10 seconds**

Total time **25 minutes**

THE EXERCISES

#	Exercise	Page
1	STATIONARY LUNGE AND CURL	p.144
2	STIFF-LEG DEADLIFT AND SHRUG	p.92
3	CHAIR DIPS	p.52
4	DIAGONAL CHOP	p.122
5	BENT ROW AND HAMMER CURL	p.82
6	SUITCASE SQUAT	p.124
7	ONE-ARM MILITARY PRESS	p.50
8	STAGGERED REVERSE FLY	p.76
9	REVERSE LUNGE WITH TWIST	p.128
10	STANDING ELBOW TO KNEE	p.98

Lower-back strength

The lower back is a vital link between your upper and lower body that's necessary for functional movements. Strengthen your lower back with these exercises to improve your coordination and become more physically efficient at all of your daily activities.

WHAT YOU NEED
Dumbbells, mat

YOUR WORKOUT

- Select the level as required by your exercise programme.
- Perform the entire sequence of exercises in order for the prescribed number of times. Use a stopwatch to follow the work and rest intervals.
- To protect your lower back from strain, keep your core engaged and maintain a flat back for all of these exercises.

THE LEVELS

LEVEL 1

Carry out the exercise sequence
2 times

Perform each exercise for
20 seconds

Rest between each exercise for
10 seconds

Total time
5 minutes

LEVEL 2

Carry out the exercise sequence
2 times

Perform each exercise for
30 seconds

Rest between each exercise for
15 seconds

Total time
7 minutes

LEVEL 3

Carry out the exercise sequence
3 times

Perform each exercise for
40 seconds

Rest between each exercise for
10 seconds

Total time
**12 minutes
30 seconds**

THE EXERCISES

1	BIRD DOG	p.88
2	GOOD MORNING	p.132
3	HIP-UPS	p.136
4	POSTERIOR SWING	p.130
5	CROSSOVER TOE TOUCH	p.114

Upper-body strength

A well-balanced upper body is crucial for proper posture. The muscles that enable you to push and pull are often weakened, lengthened, or tightened by daily habits, so use this workout to restore muscular balance to your arms, chest, and back.

WHAT YOU NEED
Dumbbells, chair, countertop

YOUR WORKOUT

- Select the level as required by your exercise programme.
- Perform the entire sequence of exercises in order for the prescribed number of times. Use a stopwatch to follow the work and rest intervals.
- For the most effective muscle recruitment, keep your focus on the muscles you are working.

THE LEVELS

LEVEL 1

Carry out the exercise sequence **2 times**

Perform each exercise for **20 seconds**

Rest between each exercise for **10 seconds**

Total time **7 minutes**

LEVEL 2

Carry out the exercise sequence **2 times**

Perform each exercise for **30 seconds**

Rest between each exercise for **15 seconds**

Total time **10 minutes**

LEVEL 3

Carry out the exercise sequence **3 times**

Perform each exercise for **40 seconds**

Rest between each exercise for **10 seconds**

Total time **17 minutes 30 seconds**

THE EXERCISES

1	ONE-ARM CHEST PRESS	p.62
2	BENT ROW AND HAMMER CURL	p.82
3	CHAIR DIPS	p.52
4	ONE-ARM SNATCH	p.86
5	CURL AND SHOULDER PRESS AND REACH	p.56
6	INCLINED PUSH-UPS	p.54
7	STAGGERED REVERSE FLY	p.76

Lower-body strength

You engage your lower body every time you squat down to pick up boxes, carry groceries, or move furniture. Perform these functional lower-body exercises to promote stability, improve strength, and prevent lower-back strains.

YOUR WORKOUT

- Select the level as required by your exercise programme.
- Perform the entire sequence of exercises in order for the prescribed number of times. Use a stopwatch to follow the work and rest intervals.
- For the most efficient lower-body workout, keep your core engaged and your back flat for all of these exercises.

THE LEVELS

LEVEL 1

Carry out the exercise sequence **2 times**

Perform each exercise for **20 seconds**

Rest between each exercise for **10 seconds**

Total time **7 minutes**

LEVEL 2

Carry out the exercise sequence **2 times**

Perform each exercise for **30 seconds**

Rest between each exercise for **15 seconds**

Total time **10 minutes**

LEVEL 3

Carry out the exercise sequence **3 times**

Perform each exercise for **40 seconds**

Rest between each exercise for **10 seconds**

Total time **17 minutes 30 seconds**

THE EXERCISES

1	LATERAL STEP-UPS	p.140
2	SUITCASE SQUAT	p.124
3	WALKING REACHING LUNGE	p.126
4	GOOD MORNING	p.132
5	REVERSE LUNGE WITH TWIST	p.128
6	HIP-UPS	p.136
7	SIDE LUNGE	p.146

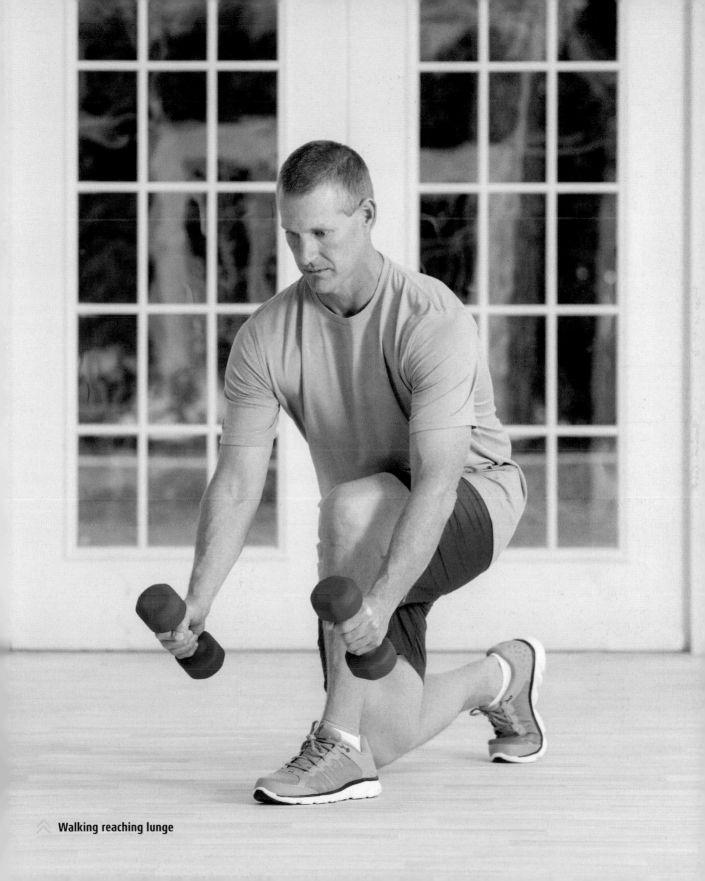

Walking reaching lunge

Low-impact aerobic

To improve your cardiovascular fitness while going easy on your joints, do this low-impact routine. This sequence of aerobic exercises places low stress on your joints while still improving your endurance and strengthening your heart.

WHAT YOU NEED
Dumbbells, wall

YOUR WORKOUT

- Select the level as required by your exercise programme.
- Perform the entire sequence of exercises in order two times. Use a stopwatch to follow the work and rest intervals.
- Perform the exercises swiftly to boost your heart rate. If you can hold a conversation during your workout, push yourself a little harder.

THE LEVELS

LEVEL 1

Carry out the exercise sequence
2 times

Perform each exercise for
15 seconds

Rest between each exercise for
15 seconds

Total time
10 minutes

LEVEL 2

Carry out the exercise sequence
2 times

Perform each exercise for
20 seconds

Rest between each exercise for
10 seconds

Total time
10 minutes

LEVEL 3

Carry out the exercise sequence
2 times

Perform each exercise for
30 seconds

Rest between each exercise for
10 seconds

Total time
13 minutes

THE EXERCISES

1	FAST FEET	p.26
2	STANDING ELBOW TO KNEE	p.98
3	POSTERIOR SWING	p.130
4	JUMPING WALL PUSH-UPS	p.66
5	SIDE-TO-SIDE	p.28
6	SEESAW ROW	p.94
7	STANDING TWIST	p.108
8	PUSH PRESS	p.60
9	MARCH IN PLACE	p.32
10	EARTHQUAKES	p.138

Cool down

This quick and effective cool down helps your body smoothly transition from exercising to a resting state. Follow the routine after every workout to slowly reduce your heart rate, prevent dizziness, and resume a normal breathing pattern.

WHAT YOU NEED
Wall, mat

YOUR WORKOUT

- After every workout, perform the entire sequence of cool-down exercises in order at least once, but repeat as necessary until you reach a resting state.
- Do not use dumbbells for any of these exercises.
- Focus on gradually lowering your heart rate, and be proud of yourself for making it through the day's workout.

THE LEVELS

ALL LEVELS

Carry out the exercise sequence at least **1 time**

Perform each exercise for **20 seconds**

Rest between each exercise for **10 seconds**

Total time **2 minutes 30 seconds**

THE EXERCISES

1	MARCH IN PLACE	p.32
2	CHEST OPENER	p.58
3	WALL ANGEL	p.84
4	UPRIGHT EXTERNAL ROTATION	p.80
5	HIP-UPS	p.136

FITNESS
PROGRAMMES

Regain your functional strength and mobility and create a healthy habit of exercise by following one of these 30-day fitness programmes. Built from the routines in the previous chapter, each programme is an easy-to-follow schedule of workouts that you can integrate into your active life.

Beginner

Every winner was once a beginner – this programme is the perfect way to begin your fitness journey. Follow the schedule and notice your body becoming stronger and more mobile as you confidently attack each day.

WORK DAYS

Begin each day with the *Warm up* (p.152). After completing the day's routine(s), finish your workout with the *Cool down* (p.179).

If any week is too strenuous, repeat that week until you feel confident enough to progress. Once you complete all four weeks, re-assess your fitness level and repeat the programme, or start the next programme.

REST DAYS

Your body needs down time to recover, so always take two rest days per week. However, you can shift the work and rest days within each week to fit your schedule.

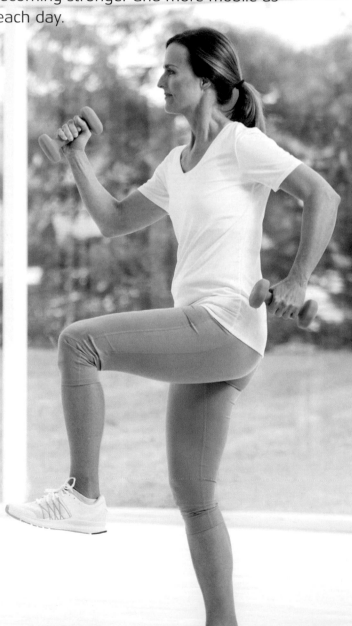

WEEK 1

WEEK 2

WEEK 3

WEEK 4

⌃ **March in place**

DAY 1	DAY 2	DAY 3	DAY 4	DAY 5	DAY 6	DAY 7
· **5-minute kick-start:** level 1 *page 153*	· **Beginner total body:** level 1 *page 156*	· **Low-intensity strength:** level 1 *page 157* · **Posture improvement:** level 1 *page 167*	· Rest	· **Low-impact aerobic:** level 1 *page 178*	· **Core strength:** level 1 *page 168*	· Rest
· **Total-body mobility:** level 1 *page 161*	· **Prehabilitation:** level 1 *page 166*	· **Beginner total body:** level 1 *page 156*	· Rest	· **Balance and stability:** level 1 *page 160*	· **Lower-back strength:** level 1 *page 174*	· Rest
· **Low-impact aerobic:** level 2 *page 178*	· **Core strength:** level 2 *page 168* · **Posture improvement:** level 1 *page 167*	· **Beginner total body:** level 2 *page 156*	· Rest	· **Balance and stability:** level 1 *page 160* · **Lower-back strength:** level 1 *page 174*	· **Total-body strength 2:** level 1 *page 173*	· Rest
· **Cardiovascular endurance:** level 1 *page 154*	· **Beginner total body:** level 2 *page 156*	· **Total-body mobility:** level 1 *page 161* · **Posture improvement:** level 1 *page 167*	· Rest	· **Low-impact aerobic:** level 2 *page 178*	· **Total-body strength 2:** level 2 *page 173*	· Rest

Intermediate

You already have a foundation of strength and stability, so break out of your comfort zone and use this programme to continue growing stronger and building a lifelong habit of functional exercise.

WORK DAYS

Begin each day with the *Warm up* (p.152). After completing the day's routine(s), finish your workout with the *Cool down* (p.179).

If any week is too strenuous, repeat that week until you feel confident enough to progress. Once you complete all four weeks, re-assess your fitness level and repeat the programme, or start the next programme.

REST DAYS

Your body needs down time to recover, so always take two rest days per week. However, you can shift the work and rest days within each week to fit your schedule.

Lawn mower row

WEEK 1

WEEK 2

WEEK 3

WEEK 4

DAY 1	DAY 2	DAY 3	DAY 4	DAY 5	DAY 6	DAY 7
· **Cardiovascular endurance:** level 2 *page 154*	· **Total-body strength 1:** level 2 *page 171*	· **Core strength:** level 2 *page 168*	· Rest	· **Calorie-burning HIIT:** level 2 *page 165*	· **Total-body strength 2:** level 2 *page 173*	· Rest
· **Lower-body strength:** level 2 *page 176*	· **Upper-body strength:** level 2 *page 175*	· **Total-body mobility:** level 2 *page 161*	· Rest	· **Cardiovascular endurance:** level 2 *page 154*	· **Calorie-burning HIIT:** level 2 *page 165*	· Rest
· **Total-body strength 1:** level 2 *page 171*	· **Balance and stability:** level 2 *page 160* · **Posture improvement:** level 2 *page 167*	· **Cross-training:** level 2 *page 162*	· Rest	· **Prehabilitation:** level 2 *page 166* · **Low-impact aerobic:** level 2 *page 178*	· **Total-body strength 2:** level 2 *page 173*	· Rest
· **Speed and agility:** level 2 *page 158*	· **Total-body mobility:** level 2 *page 161*	· **Cross-training:** level 2 *page 162*	· Rest	· **Upper-body strength:** level 2 *page 175*	· **Lower-body strength:** level 2 *page 176*	· Rest

Advanced

Speed, power, strength, balance, and coordination are all necessary components of functional movement. Push yourself with this challenging programme and achieve a high level of functional fitness.

WORK DAYS

Begin each day with the *Warm up* (p.152). After completing the day's routine(s), finish your workout with the *Cool down* (p.179).

If any week is too strenuous, repeat that week until you feel confident enough to progress. Once you complete all four weeks, repeat the programme while increasing the weight of your dumbbells and selecting the harder modifications.

REST DAYS

Your body needs down time to recover, so always take two rest days per week. However, you can shift the work and rest days within each week to fit your schedule.

WEEK 1

WEEK 2

WEEK 3

WEEK 4

⌃ **Shot-put press**

DAY 1	DAY 2	DAY 3	DAY 4	DAY 5	DAY 6	DAY 7
· **Calorie-burning HIIT:** level 3 *page 165*	· **Total-body strength 2:** level 3 *page 173*	· **Balance and stability:** level 3 *page 160* · **Posture improvement:** level 3 *page 167*	· Rest	· **Cross-training:** level 3 *page 162*	· **Core strength:** level 3 *page 168*	· Rest
· **Total-body strength 1:** level 3 *page 171*	· **Cardiovascular endurance:** level 3 *page 154*	· **Prehabilitation:** level 3 *page 166*	· Rest	· **Lower-body strength:** level 3 *page 176*	· **Upper-body strength:** level 3 *page 175*	· Rest
· **Speed and agility:** level 3 *page 158*	· **Total-body mobility:** level 3 *page 161*	· **Total-body strength 2:** level 3 *page 173*	· Rest	· **Cross-training:** level 3 *page 162*	· **Cardiovascular endurance:** level 3 *page 154*	· Rest
· **Lower-body strength:** level 3 *page 176*	· **Upper-body strength:** level 3 *page 175*	· **Calorie-burning HIIT:** level 3 *page 165*	· Rest	· **Total-body strength 1:** level 3 *page 171*	· **Speed and agility:** level 3 *page 158*	· Rest

Index

About the author

As an ISSA-certified trainer, Joshua Kozak is a seasoned leader and motivator in the fitness industry with over 15 years of experience. Through his HASfit brand, he has helped over 60 million people all over the globe get stronger and healthier with his highly effective yet simple workouts, found on HASfit.com or YouTube. Kozak's positive motivational style has earned him many accolades, including being named one of the "Top 10 Trainers on YouTube" by Google in 2014, 2015, and 2016.

Kozak is a loving father to his daughter, Alessandra, and an adoring husband to his wife, Claudia.

Author's dedication

My dear Claudia,

You sacrifice. You support. You do all of the real work. No great woman stands behind me, because you stand beside me. Thank you for keeping me humble, making me breakfast every morning, laughing at my cheesy jokes, and listening to me while I talk your ear off. You're the greatest gift the Lord could ever give me.

Joshua

Publisher's acknowledgments

DK would like to thank the following:

Models Iroy Leach, Tami Soetenga, Rachel Pfeiffer, Keith Payne, and Olga Imperial Keegan

Proofreader Laura Caddell

Indexer Celia McCoy

Bibliography

Pages 14–15
Strengthens bones J. Watkins, "Physical activity helps reduce bone loss", (extract from J. Watkins, *Structure and Function of the Musculoskeletal System, Second Edition*, Illinois, USA: Human Kinetics, 2010) Human Kinetics, http://www.humankinetics.com/excerpts/excerpts/physical-activity-helps-reduce-bone-loss; **Builds lean muscle** "Sarcopenia With Aging", WebMD Medical Reference, http://www.webmd.com/healthy-aging/guide/sarcopenia-with-aging#1; **Preserves vital joint tissues** A. Sinha, *Remedies and Cures for the Common Diseases*, New York: Page Publishing Inc., 2015; **Sharpens nervous system** "Stop falling: start saving lives and money", AgeUK, http://www.ageuk.org.uk/documents/en-gb/campaigns/stop_falling_report_web.pdf?dtrk=true; **Improves heart health and blood flow** "Cardiovascular diseases (CVDs)", World Health Organization, http://www.who.int/mediacentre/factsheets/fs317/en/; **Extends life span** S.C. Moore, A.V. Patel, C.E. Matthews et al, "Leisure Time Physical Activity of Moderate to Vigorous Intensity and Mortality: A Large Pooled Cohort Analysis", *Public Library of Science* no. 9 (11), November 2012, DOI: https://doi.org/10.1371/journal.pmed.1001335; **Improves mood and confidence** A. Pietrangelo, "Depression and Mental Health by the Numbers: Facts, Statistics, and You", Healthline, http://www.healthline.com/health/depression/facts statistics-infographic; **Increases lung function** G. Sharma and J. Goodwin, "Effect of aging on respiratory system physiology and immunology", *Clinical Interventions in Aging* no. 1 (3), September 2006, 253–260; **Boosts metabolism** G. Boston, "Basal metabolic rate changes as you age", *Washington Post*, 5 March 2013

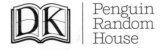

DK UK
Senior editor Kate Meeker
Senior art editor Glenda Fisher
Angliciser Victoria Heyworth-Dunne
Jacket designer Steve Marsden
Creative technical support Sonia Charbonnier
Pre-production producer Robert Dunn
Senior producer Stephanie McConnell
Managing editor Stephanie Farrow
Managing art editor Christine Keilty

DK US
Development editor Alexandra Elliott
Acquisitions editor Brook Farling
Book designer XAB Design
Art director for photography Nigel Wright
Photographer Elese Keturah Bales
Associate publisher Billy Fields
Publisher Mike Sanders

First published in Great Britain in 2017 by
Dorling Kindersley Limited
80 Strand, London, WC2R 0RL

A CIP catalogue record for this book
is available from the British Library.
ISBN: 978-0-2412-9575-5

Printed and bound in China

All images © Dorling Kindersley Limited
For further information see: www.dkimages.com

A WORLD OF IDEAS:
SEE ALL THERE IS TO KNOW

www.dk.com